Creating Sustainable Physician–Hospital Strategies

Your board, staff, or clients may also benefit from this book's insight. For more information on quantity discounts, contact the Health Administration Press Marketing Manager at (312) 424-9470.

This publication is intended to provide accurate and authoritative information in regard to the subject matter covered. It is sold, or otherwise provided, with the understanding that the publisher is not engaged in rendering professional services. If professional advice or other expert assistance is required, the services of a competent professional should be sought.

The statements and opinions contained in this book are strictly those of the author(s) and do not represent the official positions of the American College of Healthcare Executives or of the Foundation of the American College of Healthcare Executives.

12 11 10 09 08   5 4 3 2 1

Library of Congress Cataloging-in-Publication Data

Warden, Jay.
  Creating sustainable physician-hospital strategies / Jay Warden.
     p. ; cm. — (Executive essentials)
  Includes bibliographical references.
  ISBN 978-1-56793-305-5
     1. Hospital-physician relations. 2. Hospitals—Administration. I. Title. II. Series.
  [DNLM: 1. Hospital Administration—manpower. 2. Hospital Administration—standards. 3. Hospital Administrators—standards. 4. Interprofessional Relations. 5. Physicians—trends. WX 155 W265c 2009]
  RA971.9.W37 2009
  362.11068—dc22

                                                                    2008038476

The paper used in this publication meets the minimum requirements of American National Standard for Information Sciences—Permanence of Paper for Printed Library Materials, ANSI Z39.48-1984. ⊚™

Acquisitions editors: Janet Davis and Eileen Lynch; Project manager: Amanda Bove; Cover designer: Anne Locascio

Health Administration Press
A division of the Foundation of the
  American College of Healthcare Executives
1 North Franklin Street, Suite 1700
Chicago, IL 60606-3529
(312) 424-2800

Introduction

Members of the American College of Healthcare Executives, in ACHE's most recent survey, ranked "physician-hospital relations" as the #2 issue confronting hospitals, surpassed only by the issue of "financial challenges." (ACHE 2008)

The financial and competitive success of hospitals and physicians is inextricably linked, thus making physician-hospital relations one of, if not *the,* most critical components of the "financial challenges" issue cited by ACHE members. Few healthcare executives can afford *not* to focus on this book's topic. The message has been clear for nearly a decade: Find ways to collaborate with physicians for mutual growth and keep the relationships strong or watch competition chip away at profitable service lines, deplete referral sources, and impair the hospital's ability to provide needed services.

The next five years will be one of the most transformative periods for physician-hospital relationships in recent history. A number of key forces are rapidly converging to alter the nature of such relations. Issues include:

- an increasing shortage of physicians;
- soaring medical practice risk and costs;
- continued emergence of high-impact, high-cost technologies;
- shifting competition in profitable service lines; and
- changes and uncertainty on the payment and regulatory fronts.

Hospital and health system leaders must understand the pressures these issues create for physicians and commit to building the trust required for true physician-hospital partnerships. Based on such understanding and commitment, hospital executives then must identify the alignment strategies most able to address the issues, develop a fact-based physician engagement plan that balances strategic objectives with financial viability, and commit the capital and other resources required to achieve the plan.

A hospital or health system's ability to fund physician and other resource-intensive strategies is substantially dependent on its ability to raise affordable capital in the debt markets. This, in turn, is highly dependent on the strength of the organization's balance sheet, credit rating, and overall creditworthiness.

The agencies that rate debt issued by hospitals focus a significant amount of energy on analyzing physician-hospital relations. They look at

- the economics of existing and proposed physician-engagement activities, such as joint ventures and employment models, and their impact on the organization's overall financial health; and
- the negative impact to volumes and net income of poorly or unaligned physician-hospital ventures.

Notes one rating agency, "As physicians will always be an integral part of healthcare operations, their relationships with healthcare organizations—whether positive or negative—will continue to have an effect on not-for-profit credit ratings for years to come" (Standard & Poor's 2007). The development and funding of a physician-hospital plan represent a solid starting point. Strategies then must be properly implemented, monitored, and achieved. Strong healthcare organizations define indicators of an initiative's success, measure performance against these indicators, and devise and implement plans to respond to less-than-anticipated performance.

The successful execution of strategies that enable physicians to achieve their clinical and financial goals is *the* critical success factor for hospitals. Organizations that take a proactive approach will be better positioned to achieve competitive strength and the related benefits, including the ability to recruit top-ranked physicians, gain and maintain physician loyalties, and enhance revenue and market share in both inpatient and outpatient arenas.

The recommended approach to best-practice physician-hospital engagement has four steps, each of which answers a key question:

1. What do we need to know about existing physician-related trends?

2. What is our current market position and state of relations with physicians?
3. Which engagement options should we consider?
4. How do we select and implement the options and maintain a successful strategy to sustain physician-hospital alignment into the future?

Through use of a solid fact base that guides decision making, the best-practice approach balances strategic direction and financial capabilities. Applicable to all healthcare organizations—from small community hospitals to large health systems—the process ensures that the physician plan is fully integrated with the organization's overall capital, strategic, and financial plans. The result is strategies that can be implemented and sustained for win-win relationships.

CHAPTER 1

What Do We Need to Know About Existing Physician Trends?

As the primary revenue driver, physicians are critical to hospitals' ability to achieve their strategic and financial objectives. Numerous forces, however, are converging to make physician-hospital relationships challenging for many hospitals and health systems. These include staffing shortages, capacity constraints, competition from for-profit and niche providers, and increasing costs associated with the latest technology.

It is not easy for physicians either; the medical practice environment is challenging. Payments are constrained, malpractice costs are up, tests and procedures are scrutinized by payers, and 15-minute visits are often required to generate the revenue needed to sustain the practice. ▸

"Depressed and disenfranchised, physicians are responding by changing specialties, relocating to areas with better demographics and payer mix, moving as many services as possible into their offices, and looking for other ways to boost sagging income," comments one senior analyst (Goldstein 2007). A look at key trends will provide further insight into the challenges, their interrelationship, and outcomes.

PHYSICIANS' EARNINGS ARE UNDER PRESSURE

Physician incomes have been falling during the past decade. According to a study by the Center for Studying Health System Change (HSC), average overall net physician income, after adjusting for inflation, declined about 7 percent from 1995 to 2003 (Tu and Ginsburg 2006). Primary care physicians (PCPs) and surgical specialists fared worse, with a 10 percent and 8 percent decline, respectively. Medical specialists did a bit better, with only a 2 percent decrease. In contrast, workers in other professional and technical occupations experienced inflation-adjusted wage and salary increases of about 7 percent during the same period.

Flat or declining fees from Medicare, Medicaid, and private payers was the major factor cited in the HSC study for physician income stagnation or decline (Tu and Ginsburg 2006). In recent years, annual Medicare rate increases have lagged behind inflation (see Figure 1.1). Increased volume of services, particularly tests and procedures, offset some of this downward payment trend, but most physicians are experiencing significant payment issues.

Although the practice of medicine remains a highly compensated profession, the costs associated with medical school education, residency training, and deferred earnings represent significant investments that extend well beyond those of other professions. Graduates of the medical school class of 2007 who borrowed money for their education had average debt of nearly $140,000 (Association of American Medical Colleges 2007a). Physicians typically start their professional life with a high debt load.

As physicians work harder to maintain their incomes, they are making choices that have major impacts on hospital operations. These choices include consolidating hospital privileges, discontinuing the provision of call coverage or requiring sizeable pay-for-call arrangements, limiting pro bono work (including charity care and participation on

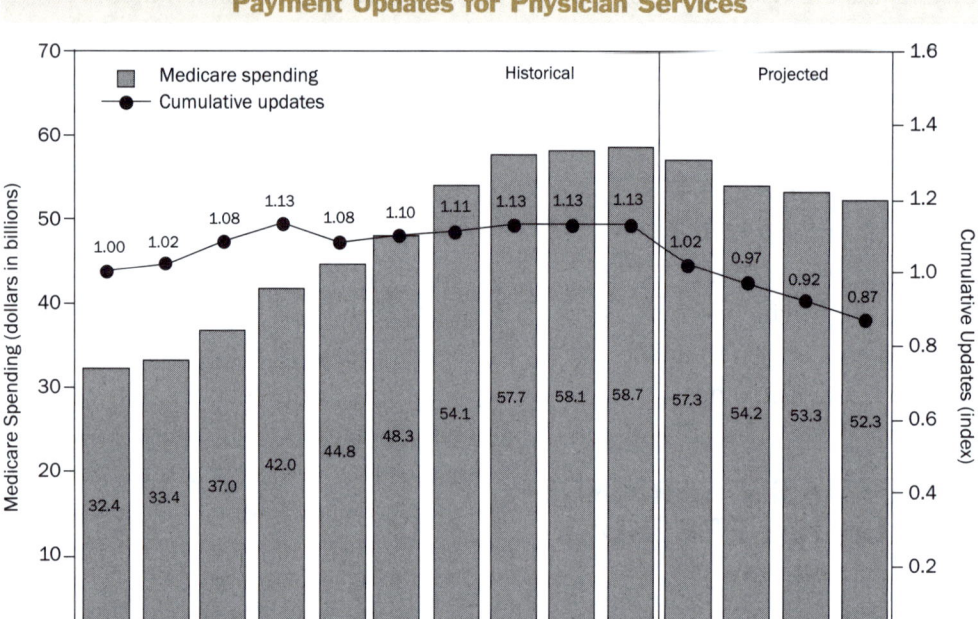

Figure 1.1. Medicare Spending and Cumulative Payment Updates for Physician Services

Source: Adapted from Medicare Payment Advisory Commission. 2008. *A Data Book: Healthcare Spending and the Medicare Program.* Washington, DC: Medicare Payment Advisory Commission.

hospital committees), and investing in ambulatory and other facilities that offer the possibility of additional income.

The latter strategy may not currently be yielding the hoped-for results, thus exacerbating the frustration of physicians who saw the development of for-profit outpatient facilities as a solution to their economic woes. After nearly a decade of revenue gains by physicians who

invested in ambulatory facilities, the physician-hospital pendulum is swinging back to a point of relative equilibrium. Consider the following:

- Physician-owned imaging facilities are experiencing substantially reduced margins since the Deficit Reduction Act (DRA) of 2005 took effect in January 2007. DRA caps Medicare Part B payments to physicians for specific imaging services.

- Physician-owned ambulatory surgery centers, which have been achieving significant success at the expense of hospital offerings in many areas of the country, experienced the first blows of reduced payments from the Centers for Medicare & Medicaid Services (CMS) in January 2008; over the next four years (2008–2011), the new payment rate, averaging approximately 65 percent of the hospital outpatient department payment rate, will be phased in for physician-owned surgery centers (Centers for Medicare & Medicaid Services 2007).

Physician entrepreneurship is hitting some regulatory and payment speed bumps as well, but continued advances in technology are enabling more and more procedures and tests to migrate from the inpatient setting to physician offices and freestanding ambulatory suites. One state hospital association comments on the results: "Rather than wait their turn for hospitals to come up with the capital and technology to accommodate their needs, some specialists choose to do business with (physician and for-profit) groups in other markets" (St. Luke's Health Initiatives and Arizona Hospital and Healthcare Association 2005).

PHYSICIAN SHORTAGES ARE GROWING

Already experienced in various locations across the country, the physician shortfall is projected to rise to 125,000 to 200,000 by 2020 (Association of American Medical Colleges 2007b). A significant proportion of active physicians are nearing retirement age and beginning to wind down practice. As indicated in Figure 1.2, one-third of practicing physicians are over age 55. The number of active physicians per 1,000 persons is declining significantly.

Gender is playing a role in physician shortages. Although female physicians represent an increasing proportion of the profession, the data indicate that women doctors desire predictable work hours and may be less likely than their male counterparts of previous decades to work long hours (Inglehart 2008). New medical school graduates of both sexes appear to place a high premium on work-life balance, and many do not wish to work 80-hour weeks (Inglehart 2008).

These trends indicate that considerably more physicians will be required to meet U.S. healthcare needs, particularly when the baby boomer population reaches its peak period of need.

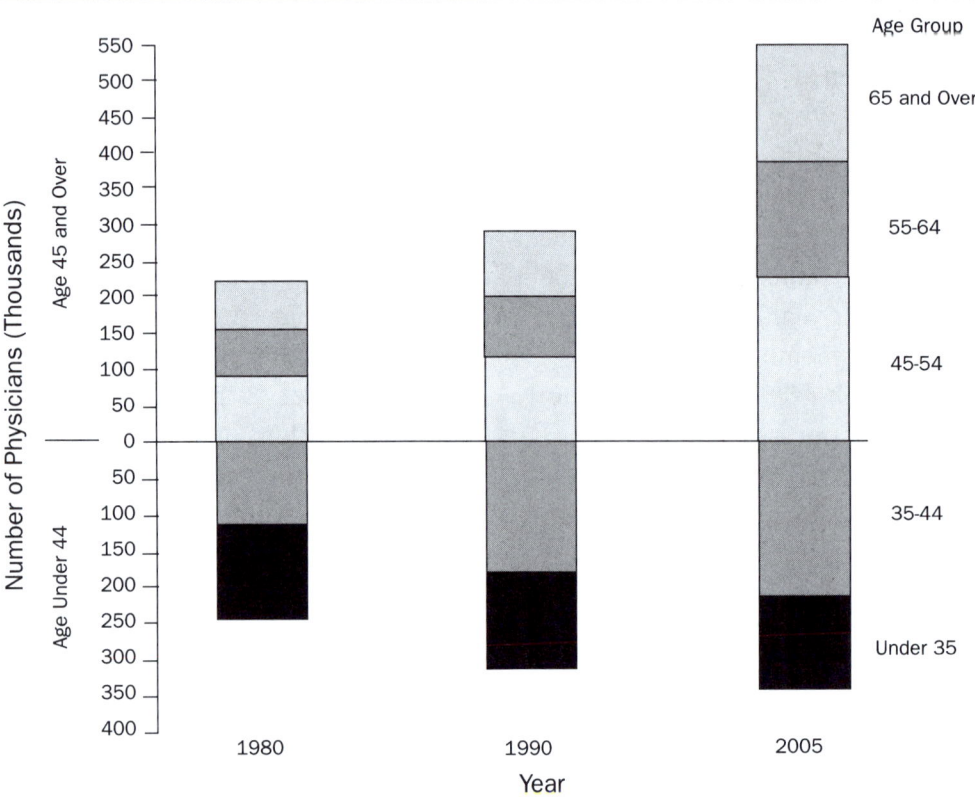

Figure 1.2. Number of Physicians by Age: 1980, 1990, and 2005

Source: American Medical Association. 2007. *Physician Characteristics and Distribution in the U.S.* Chicago: American Medical Association. Used with permission.

Unfortunately, the future physician pipeline is not adequately filled; although the U.S. population grew by more than 70 million people between 1980 and 2000, the number of medical school graduates remained 16,000 per year (Association of American Medical Colleges 2006). In 2006, the Association of American Medical Colleges recommended increasing medical school enrollment by 30 percent over the next decade—from approximately 16,500 new matriculants in 2002 to approximately 21,400 matriculants in 2015 (Association of American Medical Colleges 2006). Even with this boost, however, physician supply may very well remain below projected demand as the country's "best and brightest" steer away from the medical profession's economic challenges and choose more financially lucrative career paths.

The physician shortage is making it difficult for hospitals in many regions nationwide to recruit high-demand specialists, particularly in critical care, trauma, and emergency medicine. More than 50 percent of recently surveyed hospital chief executive officers (CEOs) described the process of recruiting physicians as "more difficult" in 2007 than in 2005. Eighty-six percent of the surveyed CEOs were recruiting physicians, and, of these, 80 percent were seeking PCPs and 74 percent were seeking specialists (Council on Physician and Nurse Supply 2007). National studies cite severe forthcoming shortages of physicians in geriatric medicine, neurosurgery, oncology, primary care, and rheumatology, among others (Association of American Medical Colleges 2007b).

PRIMARY CARE IS INCREASINGLY IMPORTANT BUT ALSO IN SCARCE SUPPLY

Given the importance of PCPs to specialty referrals, a forecasted shortage of PCPs will be particularly disrup-tive to hospitals and health systems. The following observations indicate the depth of the problem:

- The overall proportion of PCPs is declining nationally, as some seek new specialties and others retire. In 2000, 39.8 percent of physicians were PCPs; five years later, that proportion had declined to 36.7 percent (Tu and O'Malley 2007).

- Recent medical school graduates are not choosing to train in primary care specialties at the same rate as in past decades (Pham and Ginsburg 2007). For example, the proportion of medical students entering internal medicine training programs has declined to 20 percent of graduating residents in 2005 from 54 percent in 1998 (American College of Physicians 2006).

- Those physicians who are choosing an internal medicine focus are increasingly choosing hospital-based medicine because of its predictable hours. The ranks of hospitalists, a large proportion of whom are employed directly by hospitals and work defined shifts providing inpatient care, have increased dramatically since the hospitalist concept emerged a little more than decade ago. Current estimates of hospitalists working in the United States range from 12,000 to 20,000; numbers are expected to increase to 30,000 if the hospitalist model of inpatient care becomes predominant (Lindenauer et al. 2007).

- Since 1996, the supply of male PCPs relative to the U.S. population has declined 16 percent, indicating that men are choosing medical specialties and general surgery/surgical specialties over primary care. A 40 percent increase in the supply of female PCPs relative to the population has helped offset this decline (Tu and O'Malley 2007), as have international medical graduates (IMGs), who now constitute 28.3 percent of all U.S. PCPs (Starfield and Fryer 2007). As IMGs also migrate to medical specialty practice, the proportion of IMGs that practice in primary care declined to 42 percent in 2005 from 47.1 percent in 2000, but it still remains higher than the proportion of U.S.-trained physicians in primary care (Tu and O'Malley 2007).

Even more physicians are choosing technical specialties, such as radiology and anesthesiology, which offer defined hours, greater flexibil-ity, and higher incomes than internal medicine, pediatrics, and family practice.

During the capitation frenzy of the 1990s, hospitals purchased physician practices at a rapid rate, often overpaying for primary care practices. Hospitals incurred significant losses associated with practice ownership. The absence of proper productivity incentives for physicians was at least one major reason for the financial drain; physicians who became employed by hospitals simply may have worked less.

By the late 1990s, hospitals were exiting ownership arrangements in any way they could, and many organizations took their eyes off PCPs and the importance of ensuring a formal primary care strategy. To this day, some administrators and board members have strong memories of these poor decisions (and their financial results) and continue to shy away from the development of hospital-based primary care strategies.

The primary care environment has changed, however, and hospitals must now move quickly to develop and execute aggressive primary care strategies because of the following:

- Baby boomers focus on wellness and preventive care and a continuing relationship with their PCPs. Hospitals that effectively communicate with PCPs and keep them informed of care provided to their patients will win their continued loyalty.

- PCPs play a key role in controlling referrals and patient care in a pay-for-performance environment.
- With the rapid acceptance and growth of specialists who are providing a significant proportion of care to hospitalized patients, many PCPs are now spending little or no time seeing patients in the hospital. This trend weakens the loyalty and relationship between hospitals and PCPs.
- The consolidation of PCPs into larger groups outside of a hospital-owned practice is giving PCPs increasing clout because they control referrals to specialists and hospitals. This is creating new medical staff "power" dynamics.
- Many hospitals that now employ a variety of specialists, including hospitalists, intensivists, and trauma surgeons, better understand how to run physician practices and incentivize physician productivity so that they can effectively operate primary care practices at or close to a break-even level.

A PREFERENCE FOR EMPLOYMENT IS GROWING RAPIDLY

An increasing number of physicians across virtually all specialties are now seeking employment to lower their exposure to risk; to protect themselves from rising costs related to malpractice insurance, leases, and support staff; and to achieve a better work-life balance. Because of lifestyle issues, Generation X physicians (born between 1965 and 1980) may be particularly interested in hospital-based employment. These physicians tend to be more risk averse and look at medicine as a job. As health plans increasingly require group affiliation for participation, independent physicians of all ages may also consider employment in a hospital-affiliated group practice to be an attractive alternative.

Employment of physicians by hospitals, particularly in high-demand, low-supply specialties, can mitigate staff-shortage issues. Beyond increasing the hospital's ability to deliver needed services, physician employment enables the hospital to direct the physician's time to activities that may have a substantial impact on cost-effective service delivery, clinical quality improvement, and financial performance.

As described further in Chapter 3, many hospitals are starting to recognize physician employment as a proactive strategy to minimize risks, grow market share, and gain increased physician participation (see Sidebar 1.1).

CONCLUDING COMMENTS

Given physician income pressures and shortages and the growing importance of primary care and hospital-based employment, we look next at how to take the pulse of a hospital's physician relations by conducting a physician audit—the second phase in the recommended approach to physician-hospital engagement.

SIDEBAR 1.1

Factors Contributing to Growth in Popularity of Physician Employment

For Physicians
- Work-life balance/flexible hours
- Protection from rising practice costs, including malpractice insurance, leases, and support staff
- Zero up-front investment means lower risk to move to a new location
- As single and multispecialty groups grow and proliferate, independent physicians find themselves needing to choose a partner or risk being shut out of health plans

For Hospitals
- Ensures provision of services in high-demand, low-supply specialties
- Covers the emergency department, which may be short staffed as a result of growth in trauma programs and the fear of losing valued specialists who threaten to drop hospital privileges if they have to continue to take call for "unassigned" patients
- A proactive strategy to grow market share and minimize risks

Source: Kaufman, Hall & Associates, Inc. Used with permission.

CHAPTER 2

What Is Our Current Market Position and State of Physician Relations?

The road hospitals traveled to engage physicians used to be a fairly straight one: Open the hospital's doors; provide patient beds, quality nursing care, and technology; and physicians could be expected to refer the patients required for the hospital's ongoing competitive financial performance.

That means of way-finding is decidedly over. Constrained reimbursement, increased competition, higher costs, and rapidly advancing technology have made more modern navigational systems mandatory. To achieve successful physician-hospital relations in the present healthcare environment, hospitals must have detailed knowledge about their ▶

current whereabouts, define their desired end goal, and then progress toward that goal, often using multiple paths.

Multiyear planning for physician strategies—most commonly cited as five-year planning—is critical. So too are projections that prove the financial efficacy of these strategies. The absence of such planning and projections discredits a hospital or health system's physician plan. A comprehensive assessment of an organization's current strategic and financial position in its physician market provides the framework for understanding challenges and opportunities (see Sidebar 2.1). From this knowledge flows a set of critical goals or objectives that enable the organization to meet its mission *and* maintain competitive financial performance.

A structured assessment approach is highly recommended. Best-practice plans are based on strategic and market realities, so comprehensive data are required. Hospital and health system leaders must do their homework. The assessment process is cumulative. Numbers in isolation may not be critical, but the combination of data reveals the big picture about an organization's performance in its competitive environment.

SIDEBAR 2.1

Elements of a Comprehensive Physician Audit

1. Strategic market position assessment (demographics, utilization/demand, market share, competition on a specialty or service-line basis)
2. Physician market structure (supply/demand, dynamics)
3. Medical staff profile (age, group, specialty dependency, splitter analysis—i.e., analysis of physicians who refer patients to multiple hospitals)
4. Physician utilization and financial analysis (admissions/case volume)
5. Current physician-management relations, based on comprehensive physician and management interviews
6. Specific competitive activities by physicians
7. Existing physician-hospital arrangements (strategic, financial, information technology)

Source: Kaufman, Hall & Associates, Inc. Used with permission.

Numerous variables are essential to building the required quantitative fact base. Trends, which show track record and momentum, are important, in addition to annual numbers. A description of information that should be tracked and trended follows.

CONDUCTING A THOROUGH PHYSICIAN AUDIT

The physician audit begins with a strategic market position assessment, which establishes the characteristics of the environment in which the hospital operates.

Strategic Market Position Assessment

This assessment answers the following questions:

- Which market(s) does the organization serve?
- What are the current and projected future characteristics of the population and the local economy in these market(s)?
- What is the payer mix in the market(s)?

- What is the organization's market share? How has this changed over time?
- What changes are anticipated in demand for healthcare services in the market(s)? How will changes in demographics and emerging technologies affect future demand for hospital services?
- Which service lines will grow the fastest and why? Which services lines will shrink and why?
- What is the physician and other for-profit and not-for-profit competition on a specialty-by-specialty and/or service-line basis?
- How are ambulatory surgery centers or specialty hospitals affecting the hospital's business?

Although organizations often identify primary and secondary market service areas, delineation of the market service area by cluster groupings (see Figure 2.1) can provide a more complete understanding of the area. It considers such factors as patient origin, population demographics, natural/geographic boundaries, and retail trade and other patterns.

Relevant demographic data include current and projected population, age and gender distribution, and median household income. In

Figure 2.1. Cluster-based Market Service Area Definition

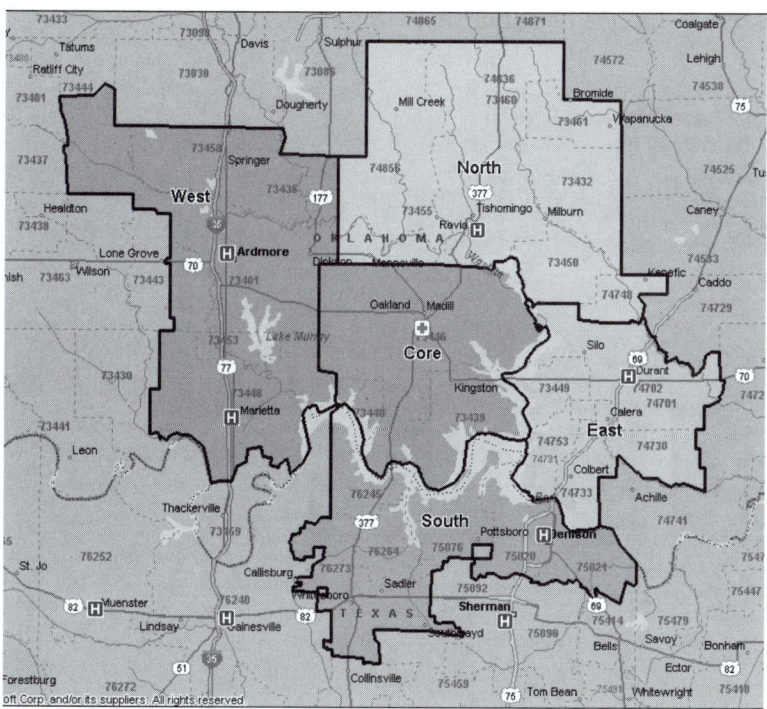

Source: Kaufman, Hall & Associates, Inc. Used with permission.

any given market, one or two of these elements could assume key importance because of trends that suggest good growth or weak socio-economics. Payer mix (overall and by service line) is an increasingly big driver of performance. The mix of government payers could be a positive or negative for the hospital depending on other factors, such as the provider/private insurer dynamic and balance of power. Market share, overall and by service line, indicates how the organization is positioned in the community. For example, Figure 2.2 shows that the market for surgical services in Hospital A's service

area is highly fragmented. However, it also shows that Hospital A is one of the three hospitals that achieve significant market share in highly profitable neurosurgery and cardiac surgery programs.

Market share analysis combined with analysis of profitability by service line provides a clearer picture of the hospital's current position and helps identify where a hospital might wish to focus in the future. Figure 2.3 is a profitability/market share matrix. It shows that the profiled hospital achieves a considerable proportion of its revenue from one service line (in quadrant II), which

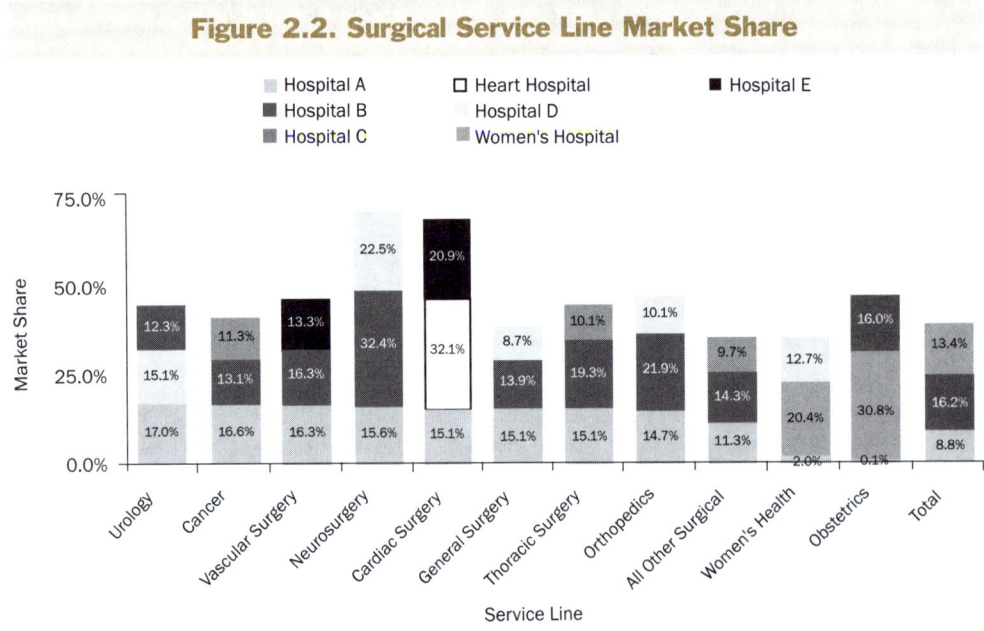

Figure 2.2. Surgical Service Line Market Share

Source: Kaufman, Hall & Associates, Inc. Used with permission.

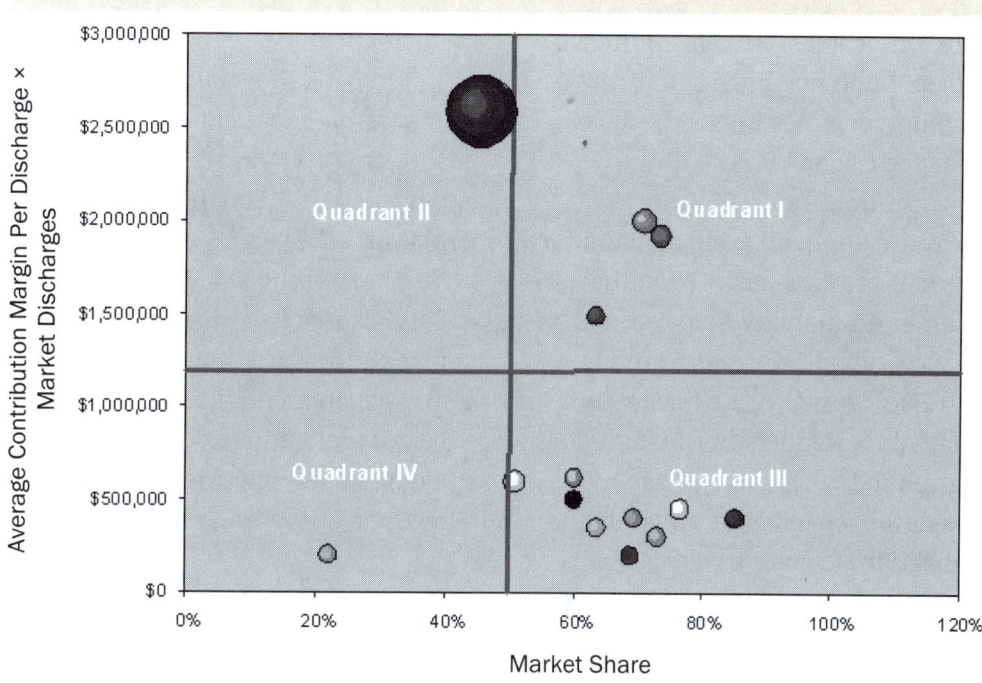

Figure 2.3. Service Line Contribution and Market Share

Source: Kaufman, Hall & Associates, Inc. Used with permission.

could make the hospital vulnerable to changes in this service line. The hospital might wish to develop strategies to defend and boost current market share for service lines in quadrant I.

Inpatient competition by service line from hospital and nonhospital competitors should be assessed carefully. An analysis of the hospital's competitive strengths, weaknesses, opportunities, and threats (a SWOT analysis) by service line can be helpful. How have competitor hos-

pitals affected the hospital's medical staff and employed physician ranks? Detailed competitor profiles can be developed from public and commercial sources. Although more challenging, organizations should also collect and track data related to outpatient market share, since physicians are often direct competitors in this arena. Some hospitals have strong, well-designed decision support systems that enable planners to thoroughly assess the organization's current outpatient business based on patient-level data. Outpatient market data from external sources, such as state or local departments of health, official bond documents, and subscription commercial sources, can enhance the analysis.

Utilization trends indicate the increasing or decreasing demand for services in years past. Given the variation in profitability by payer and/or service, not all utilization growth is "good" growth, so a review of utilization numbers in isolation does not tell the whole story. Case mix should be looked at as an adjunct to utilization. Is good payer/case mix growth occurring (i.e., insured and high acuity) or is bad payer/case mix growth occurring (i.e., nonpaying or low-paying and low acuity)?

Demand projections estimate the future market size and opportunities for specific service lines within specific market areas. Information on what competitors are doing is critical here. Use projections should provide details related to demand by specific service lines, clusters, and/or payer levels. An organization must be able to generate reliable volume demand projections that are grounded in market realities. Such projections enable the hospital to model, evaluate, and prioritize strategic growth initiatives and ef-

fectively manage the organization's long-term competitive market and financial position.

To project and evaluate the hospital's baseline inpatient demand for healthcare services, staff will need to develop the following (York and Benjamin 2008):

- Service area use rates by geography and service line
- Service area volume projections by geography and service line
- Organization-specific volume projections at the same level of detail

Figure 2.4 illustrates the process.

To complete the picture, planners often project demand for ancillary inpatient and outpatient services using an approach focused on internal data. This approach applies population, utilization rate impact, and overall market share increase assumptions to baseline data.

High-quality software tools enable planners to seamlessly integrate multiple data sources, such as commercially available data and internal data, to produce projection results by service line and/or geographic area. Projections must be based on assumptions that are plausible, defensible, and in line with past actual performance.

Figure 2.4. A Practical Approach to Projecting Baseline Inpatient Demand

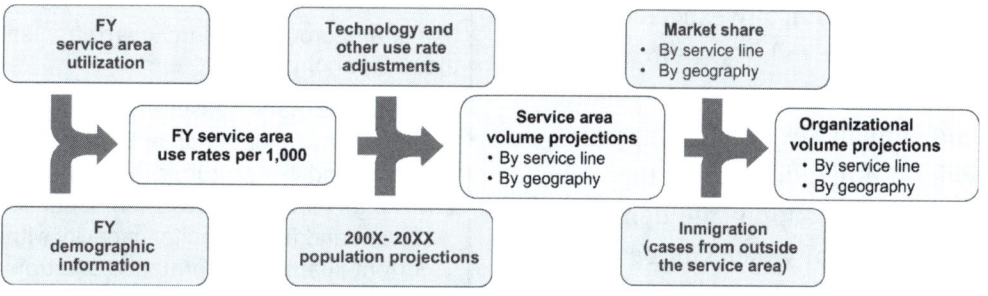

Source: Kaufman, Hall & Associates, Inc. Used with permission.

On completion of a thorough assessment of strategic market position, a hospital or health system can identify financially attractive markets and services lines for growth and can determine specific volume targets. For example, a hospital might be able to say the following:

Orthopedics, general surgery, and obstetrics represent our most attractive inpatient service lines for growth in our core-cluster market area. Specific volume added by each is projected to be A, B, and C, resulting in overall projected top-line revenue growth of $X. Imaging and women's health represent our most attractive outpatient service lines for growth in our core and northern cluster market areas. Specific volume added by each is projected to be A and B, resulting in an overall top-line revenue growth projection of $X.

Sidebar 2.2 highlights core components of growth planning.

Physician Market Structure

This analysis is the second major piece of the comprehensive physician audit. A hospital's medical staff development department or business planning staff commonly conducts studies related to physician supply and demand by specialty in the hospital's service area. This analysis is critical to ensuring that the hospital understands the number of physicians in each specialty needed to effectively serve its market. The analysis also ensures the demonstration of community need for a given specialty, which the hospital is required to complete to provide the recruitment assistance or income guarantees typically expected by physicians in today's environment.

The U.S. Department of Health and Human Services (HHS) provides a utilization-based approach to physician supply and demand, the models of which can be helpful to individual hospitals. The HHS physician-demand model combines population projections, insurance distributions, and physician-per-population ratios (see Figure 2.5). Many state medical societies also conduct similar studies. A hospital's strategic market position analysis should provide relevant demographic, payer, and physician-per-population data on a hospital-specific basis.

SIDEBAR 2.2

Core Components of Growth Planning

Use of a rigorous, systematic growth planning process includes these four components:

- A *strategic market assessment* builds an in-depth and accurate understanding of the organization's market position, key market trends, and likely future developments.
- A *capital capacity assessment* identifies the organization's current and future capital capacity within the limits of its current financial performance and trajectory. A combined look at the capital capacity assessment and the strategic market assessment defines the organization's financial and market realities, considering limitations and opportunities.
- *Growth strategy development* defines achievable strategies given market and financial realities. Strategies may focus on organic initiatives that extend programs and services, physician alignment initiatives, new market entry, and acquisitions or consolidation, among others, or a combination of such initiatives.
- The *financial impact analysis* tests potential strategies or their combinations to assess financial outcomes. Sensitivity or scenario analysis enables organizations to assess the risks underlying key performance variables.

Source: Kaufman, Hall & Associates, Inc. Used with permission.

Figure 2.5. Overview of a Physician Demand Model

Population projections by age, sex, and location	×	Insurance distribution by age, sex, and location	×	Physician-per-population ratios by age, sex, location, insurance, and physician specialty	=	Physician requirements by population characteristics and physician specialty

Source: U.S. Dept. of Health and Human Services. 2006. *Physician Supply and Demand: Projections to 2020.* Washington, DC: Health Resources and Services Administration.

Physician demographics (such as age and gender), specialty, and productivity have important supply implications. For example, age can be correlated with retirement probability and annual hours worked. Trends related to average number of patients seen and work relative value units per full-time equivalent affect projections of physician supply by specialty. The growth and aging of the population, medical insurance trends, technological advances, nonphysician clinicians, and policy changes can exert a significant impact on demand for physician services.

During this portion of the physician audit, hospitals should ask and answer the following questions:

■ How will new technology and changes in medical staff makeup affect the supply of and demand for care?

■ What level of demand will the hospital experience for physicians in shortage specialties, such as emergency care, trauma care, and neurology?

■ How is the hospital positioned relative to primary care groups that drive specialist referrals and hospital admissions?

Figure 2.6 illustrates one hospital's analysis of near-term supply and demand needs for primary care physicians (PCPs). To project demand, the hospital used three physician-to-population ratio methodologies based on insurance payment approach—traditional, blended, and managed care. The analysis indicates that the hospital should launch a

Figure 2.6. Sample Supply-Demand Study: Primary Care Physicians

Specialty	2007 Supply	2010 Market Share-Based Demand			2008–2010 Recruitment		
		Traditional	Blended	Managed Care	Traditional	Blended	Managed Care
Family Medicine	36.7	42.4	35.2	28.0	6.7	(0.5)	(7.7)
Internal Medicine	10.6	35.0	29.1	23.1	26.4	20.5	14.5
Pediatrics	10.0	14.8	12.2	9.7	4.8	2.2	(0.3)
Primary Care Total	**57.3**	**92.2**	**76.5**	**60.8**	**37.9**	**22.2**	**6.5**

Source: Kaufman, Hall & Associates, Inc. Used with permission.

significant recruitment effort to attract internal medicine physicians, but it is oversupplied with family medicine physicians.

Physician workforce assessments are more critical now than ever, so leaders should ensure thorough work on this issue.

The dynamics and organization of physicians in the market also warrant study. A medical school or a specialty hospital, for example, attracts specialized practitioners to the area. The presence of strong organized medical groups, whether primary care or specialty care in focus, will affect recruitment and retention initiatives. This topic is addressed later in the Current Physician-Management Relations section.

Medical Staff Profile/ Physician Utilization and Financial Analysis

These pieces of the physician audit assess key characteristics of the physician staff, such as age, specialty, group, admitting patterns, and physician and specialty contribution to hospital revenue. They help identify recruitment needs, physician referral patterns, hospital dependence on physicians in specific specialties, and profitability by provider and specialty.

Figure 2.7 illustrates one hospital's analysis of the top-attending physicians on its medical staff. Of its 160 medical staff physicians, the top 15 physicians—8 of whom are obstetricians/gynecologists—bring in 35 percent of the total cases. This indicates the hospital's heavy reliance on a limited number of physicians to attend inpatient cases. The average age of the top physicians is nearly 50, suggesting the need to recruit physicians to replace those nearing retirement.

Figure 2.8 shows similar results for another hospital, but data on each specialty's inpatient discharges, inpatient contribution margin, and average contribution margin per discharge are also provided. Such data enhance an organization's ability to identify vulnerabilities, dependencies, and risk of losing profitable business to competition.

The makeup of the medical staff in terms of group affiliations is also important. Are there large, multispecialty or single-specialty groups in the core market, or do small groups and solo practitioners predominate? Often, these data will be specialty specific—for example, there might be one large orthopedics group, but pediatricians are primarily solo practitioners. Group formation is often a function of market and payer dynamics.

Figure 2.7. Top Attending Physicians at Sample Hospital

Rank	Physician	Specialty	Age	Number of Cases in Fiscal Year 2007
1	A	General internal medicine	56	423
2	B	Obstetrics/gynecology	65	337
3	C	Hospitalist	41	333
4	D	Obstetrics/gynecology	63	331
5	E	Obstetrics/gynecology	56	298
6	F	Obstetrics/gynecology	45	296
7	G	Hospitalist	38	289
8	H	Family practice	43	280
9	I	Obstetrics/gynecology	37	278
10	J	Surgery, general	51	275
11	K	Obstetrics/gynecology	60	273
12	L	Nephrology	57	253
13	M	General internal medicine	35	246
14	N	Obstetrics/gynecology	61	243
15	O	Obstetrics/gynecology	37	224
Top 15 Total			49.7 (average)	4,379
Other			48.6 (average)	8,112
TOTAL			48.7 (average)	12,491

Source: Kaufman, Hall & Associates, Inc. Used with permission.

Information about hospital-based physicians, including anesthesiologists, emergency physicians, pathologists, radiologists, hospitalists, interventionalists, and others, is also critical. Do these physicians work under an exclusive agreement with the hospital (as a part of the group or on an individual basis), or do they also provide services in potentially competitive inpatient or outpatient facilities?

Current Physician-Management Relations

This portion of the audit assesses the physician-management culture and the level of physician satisfaction and loyalty the hospital currently

Figure 2.8. Medical Staff Analysis for Sample Hospital

Attending Physician Specialty	Number on Staff at Hospital 1	Splitters to Hospital 2	Percent Splitters to Hospital 2	Number on Staff at Hospital 2 and Not Hospital 1	Average Age	Inpatient Discharges at Hospital 1 in Fiscal Year 2007	Inpatient Contribution Margin at Hospital 1 ($000s) in Fiscal Year 2007	Average Contribution Margin per Discharge ($000s) in Fiscal Year 2007
Primary Care								
Family Practice	34	24	71%	3	44.6	1,257	3,259.9	2.6
Internal Medicine	35	23	66%	1	48.7	2,728	7,737.0	2.8
Pediatrics	4	3	75%	13	52.8	26	57.5	2.2
Subtotal	73	50	68%	17	47.0	4,011	11,054.4	2.8
Specialist								
Cardiology	29	25	86%	0	49.0	1,944	8,079.5	4.2
Cardiovascular/ Thoracic Surgery	9	6	67%	0	51.2	318	1,876.8	5.9
Gastroenterology	9	9	100%	0	52.7	635	2,533.5	4.0
General Surgery	10	10	100%	1	50.0	681	3,996.5	5.9
Nephrology	11	10	91%	0	46.3	321	854.6	2.7
Neurology	5	4	80%	1	54.0	15	54.9	3.7
Neurosurgery	4	4	100%	2	49.0	218	1,716.1	7.9
Oncology	10	10	100%	0	49.3	504	2,278.5	4.5
Orthopedic Surgery	15	10	67%	1	45.5	492	2,676.4	5.4
Otorhinolaryngology	5	5	100%	1	53.2	19	94.0	4.9
Physical Medicine/ Rehabilitation	3	3	100%	1	51.0	93	578.5	6.2
Plastic Surgery	4	4	100%	0	56.3	69	435.1	6.3
Podiatry	7	6	86%	1	43.7	31	227.3	7.3
Pulmonary Medicine	6	6	100%	1	47.8	238	1,061.4	4.5
Urology	11	11	100%	0	47.0	319	1,178.9	3.7
All Other	34	21	62%	29	52.0	142	1,031.0	7.3
Subtotal	172	144	84%	38	49.5	6,039	28,673.0	4.7
Hospital-Based								
Anesthesiology	7	0	0%	10	52.9	0	0.0	0.0
Emergency Medicine	9	0	0%	13	47.0	3	8.5	2.8
Pathology	3	0	0%	5	51.7	0	0.0	0.0
Radiology	8	0	0%	5	58.9	25	86.3	3.5
Subtotal	27	0	0%	33	55.3	28	94.8	3.4
Total	272	194	71%	88	49.1	10,078	39,822.2	4.0

Source: Kaufman, Hall & Associates, Inc. Used with permission.

achieves. Numerous factors are central to understanding the hospital's strengths and vulnerabilities relative to physician relations.

A *historical review* is often a good place to start. How and when was the medical staff formed? Did a large medical group establish a doctor's hospital, or did the hospital begin with an all-volunteer or private medical staff? Other considerations include:

- Past hospital mergers that could have affected or still affect medical staff dynamics;
- History of previous leadership teams' relationships with physicians;
- Past physician organizations, such as a physician-hospital organization (PHO) or an independent practice arrangement that may have affected physicians' current perspective; and
- Other marketplace dynamics, such as competitor activities and the formation or dissolution of groups.

Physician representation in *organizational governance* should be reviewed. What is the history of physician participation on the hospital's board? How are physicians selected for board participation, and what is the level of physician involvement on key board committees and in decision making? When physicians have a large capital request, do they work through board structures or directly through executive leadership?

A review of physician participation in other roles, such as on capital committees, clinical advisory panels, and strategic planning and decision-making groups, is also important. Sidebar 2.3 outlines relevant indicators of physician leadership, medical staff involvement, and medical staff dynamics.

Information about the hospital's *physician support infrastructure* can shed light on activities that may contribute to or detract from positive physician-hospital relations.

Does the hospital have a formal physician relations staff? No hospital should consider itself too small for such a staff. How many staff members are available, and what are their goals, roles, and activities? Do they visit physician offices, and, if so, how many times per week or per month? What process does the staff use to identify, resolve, and communicate resolution of issues or concerns raised by physicians? What are the metrics of physician relations success, how are they monitored, and how are results addressed as needed? Are the CEO, COO, CFO, and physician leaders spending time on physician relations daily?

Other elements of physician infrastructure support include

- the medical staff office, whose scope of activities and number of staff and roles can make a significant difference to hospital-physician relations; and
- medical staff development, which may include annual medical staff planning, dedicated staff to identify physician recruitment needs, and on-staff or contracted physician recruiters.

Some hospitals and health systems, particularly academic medical centers, offer physicians research and education support in the form of staff and/or funding.

Many hospitals employ hospitalists, intensivists, and nurse practitioners to manage patient care and procedure needs. Is the hospitalist program perceived as a net positive by PCPs? Is the hospital employing such physicians and nurses to help treat uninsured patients and to alleviate physicians' on-call and financial burden?

<table>
<tr><td style="background:#9a7d3c;color:white">SIDEBAR 2.3</td></tr>
</table>

Indicators of Physician Leadership and Medical Staff Dynamics

Physician Leadership Indicators
- Executive physician leadership roles (chief medical officer, vice president of medical affairs, chief quality officer)
- Medical staff leadership roles (medical staff officer, medical executive committee member)
- Medical department director roles
- Recruitment, training, and development of physician leaders (episodic vs. regular)
- Informal physician leadership development

Level of Medical Staff Involvement
- Frequency of meetings
- Attendance requirements
- Communication vehicles
- Participation of hospital management (CEO, chief financial officer [CFO], chief operating officer [COO])
- Nature of interaction between medical staff and hospital administration

Medical Staff Dynamics
- Competition between specialties/groups
- Trust/distrust between physicians and between physicians and hospital management
- Perceptions of unfair decisions made by hospital management that favor certain physicians or specialties over others

Source: Kaufman, Hall and Associates, Inc. Used with permission.

In-depth interviews with physicians conducted by a third party can capture a significant amount of valuable and actionable information regarding physician-hospital relations. Sidebar 2.4 provides a sample of "themes and hot spots" gleaned through interviews with physicians employed by or affiliated with a large academic medical center.

Sample Themes and Issues Identified Through Physician Interviews

- Physicians have a strong loyalty to the medical center and believe in its teaching and charitable missions. The medical center is clearly seen as the physician's choice for partnership in the region.
- Physicians have a keen interest in understanding the medical center's vision and its impact on their practice and the community.
- Physicians generally feel underrepresented in medical center decision making at the governance level and the service-line level.
- Physicians feel that the medical center is "afraid" to upset private practice physicians, so the organization often defers (sometimes indefinitely) decisions that even private practice physicians acknowledge should be made.
- Faculty physicians would like to be treated in the same manner as private practitioners (instead of being required to take a back seat).
- A sound, consistent policy and transparency regarding pay-for-call arrangements are needed.
- All physicians want an electronic medical record system as soon as possible. Communication back to PCPs is unacceptable, and the medical center is perceived as being way behind in information technology (IT) sophistication.
- Anesthesiologists are severely hampering surgeons from doing more cases at times that are convenient for surgeons and patients. Surgeons universally expect the medical center to fix this and are frustrated that it has not been addressed.

Source: Kaufman, Hall & Associates, Inc. Used with permission.

Specific Competitive Activities by Physicians

Although addressed generally as part of the strategic market position assessment, direct competition from physicians should be fully evaluated. As financial challenges increase for all healthcare providers, competition for profitable services, such as ambulatory surgery, imaging, cardiology, oncology, and orthopedic surgery, has intensified. As described in Chapter 1, eager to supplement stagnant incomes, and often supplied with capital from developers and others, physicians are opening for-profit specialty hospitals and ambulatory diagnostic and treatment centers in many regions of the country, particularly in states without certificate-of-need regulations. Able to attract well-insured patients, these centers often draw patients from the hospitals' most profitable service areas. Sidebar 2.5 provides core assessment elements.

Current Physician-Hospital Arrangements

This final element of a comprehensive physician audit is the assessment of existing economic and strategic arrangements between the hospital and physicians. Knowledge about current arrangements enables the development of viable future arrangements. Hospitals should develop a list of such arrangements and ensure that they have detailed knowledge of the policies, issues, financial terms, and strategic and financial results of each.

IT is an important element of this portion of the audit. How are physicians connected to the organization—for example, through electronic health record (EHR) or electronic medical record (EMR) systems, picture archiving and communication systems, computerized physician order entry, or electronic prescribing systems? Does connectivity enable physicians to obtain information in their offices and homes and in multiple inpatient and outpatient settings? As described in Chapter 3, hospital-physician collaboration in the area of IT can yield significant mutual benefits related to quality of care, care outcomes, and customer service. What are the strengths and weaknesses of the current systems? Does such connectivity meet physician and hospital needs?

Table 2.1 summarizes physician strategies used by more than 300 surveyed hospitals and the perceived effectiveness of such strategies.

CONCLUDING COMMENTS

After completing the comprehensive strategic analysis and physician audit described here, healthcare leaders will be better equipped to explore the full range of physician-hospital engagement options, which is the topic of Chapter 3.

Table 2.1. Most Frequently Used Strategies by Effectiveness Rating

Strategy	High Effectiveness Rating	Respondents Using Strategy
Employ a vice president of medical affairs (or equivalent leader)	74%	73%
Provide financial support for recruitment to independent physician practices	72%	83%
Actively involve physicians in planning and developing clinical service lines or centers of excellence	66%	83%
Employ primary care physicians	65%	72%
Conduct formal individual/group interviews with physicians to identify their issues and concerns	63%	78%
Implement clinical information systems that provide physicians with ready access to clinical information when they are outside the hospital	61%	73%
Pay physicians a stipend for medical directorships	54%	67%
Pay for leadership development activities for current and future physician leaders	53%	77%
Have a written medical staff development plan that outlines goals/strategies related to physician recruitment	59%	72%

Source: McGowan, R.A. and A.S. MacNulty. 2005. "Strategies for Strengthening Physician-Hospital Alignment: A National Study," Noblis (formerly Mitretek Systems, Inc.), Chicago: Society for Healthcare Marketing and Strategy Development. Used with permission.

Which Engagement Options Should We Consider?

The analysis of strategic position and the physician audit, as described in Chapter 2, enable hospital leaders to identify attractive markets and service lines for development and to assess current physician relationships in these and other areas. The next process is to identify physician-hospital engagement options that enable the organization to maintain or build its position in the markets, as specified in the organization's strategic plan. Hospitals and health systems typically employ a multitude of options, depending upon strategic priorities, competition, selected service lines, physician organization, and other factors. Education about options is critical; the hospital's entire ▶

leadership team and board of directors must be on the same page in this regard. Sidebar 3.1 outlines core elements of leadership education.

Professional associations and other industry groups provide seminars that can be helpful starting points (see Sidebar 3.2). Practical guidance from case examples and lessons learned from hospitals and health systems can be particularly valuable.

If hospital leaders are not already well versed in physician-hospital collaboration law, they need to be educated soon. Federal and state laws and regulations related to anti-kickback, Stark/self-referral, and tax exemption are complex and have a significant effect on what arrangements can and cannot be made with physicians. The laws and regulations are a moving target, so it is important for leadership to stay on top of changes. Recent implementation of Stark III is casting additional regulatory scrutiny on a number of specific options not covered in this publication, including per-click arrangements and "under arrangement" lease deals. Leaders should know enough to recognize when expert legal or tax counsel is needed. Given the rapidity of developments and adverse consequences of improperly structured arrangements, counsel is generally required early in the exploration process.

Although a detailed description of each engagement option is beyond this book's scope, key information for selected strategies is provided here. The options are presented approximately in order of the strength of physician-hospital integration

---

SIDEBAR 3.1

Physician-Hospital Strategies: Core Elements of Leadership Education

- Overview of physician-hospital engagement options
- Assessment of hospital's current market position
- Results of current physician audit
- Laws and regulations affecting alignment options
- National/state/local issues affecting options
- Key statistics, case studies, examples of strategies used in comparable markets
- Strategic- and mission-based engagement options

Source: Kaufman, Hall & Associates, Inc. Used with permission.

SIDEBAR 3.2

Selected Organizations Offering Physician-Hospital Strategy Topics

- American College of Healthcare Executives (www.ache.org)
- American College of Physician Executives (www.acpe.org)
- American Hospital Association (AHA; www.aha.org)
- Beard Group (www.beardgroup.com)
- The Governance Institute (www.governanceinstitute.com)
- Healthcare Financial Management Association (www.hfma.org)
- Healthcare Strategy Institute (www.healthcarestrategy.com)
- Health Forum (an AHA company) (www.healthforum.com)
- Society for Healthcare Strategy and Market Development (an AHA-affiliated group) (www.shsmd.org)

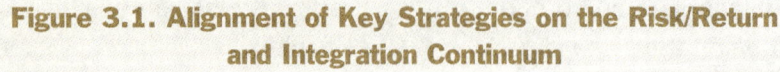

Figure 3.1. Alignment of Key Strategies on the Risk/Return and Integration Continuum

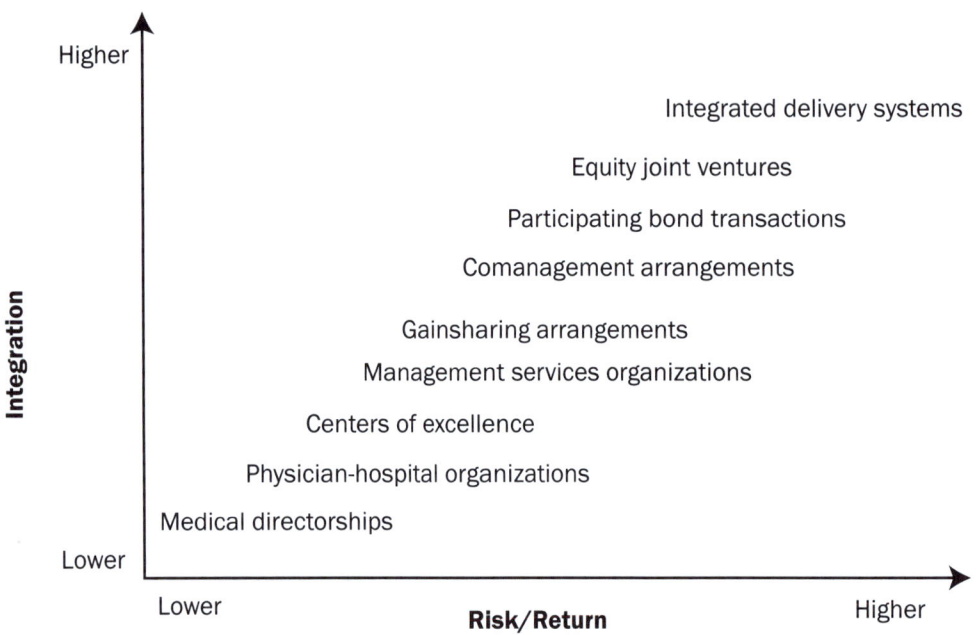

Source: Kaufman, Hall & Associates, Inc. Used with permission.

offered by each and their risk and return potential (see Figure 3.1). Table 3.1 highlights their advantages and disadvantages.

PHYSICIAN PARTICIPATION ON HOSPITAL BOARDS AND COMMITTEES

This strategy's use by all hospitals and health systems is mandatory now and into the future. Physician input to strategic direction and participation in decision making are critical to the successful implementation of initiatives in all clinical areas and to overall organizational performance.

Most hospitals and health systems have physicians with fiduciary and voting privileges on their boards. According to data from the Governance Institute, physicians on average compose nearly 20 percent of boards (see Sidebar 3.3). This proportion undoubtedly reflects the now-defunct 20 percent limit the Internal Revenue

Table 3.1. Physician–Hospital Engagement Options

Strategies	Strength of Economic Alignment	Advantages	Disadvantages
Physician input through boards and committees	Historically low, but increasing	Low cost; low risk	Longer-term benefits; no or little economic alignment
Medical directorships	Low	Flexible; can include as many physicians as necessary	Can create political conflicts; requires physician time commitment
Forgivable loans	Low	Flexible as long as there is demonstrated need	Short-lived; no guarantees of loyalty or collaboration
Information technology linkage	Medium	Easy to "touch" many physicians	Costly
Physician-hospital organizations	Medium	Some economic alignment	Loyalty is to the contracts, not the other party
Centers of excellence or clinical institutes	Medium	Ties physicians to program; improves service offering	Little economic alignment unless combined with another strategy
Management services organizations	Medium	Ties hospital to physicians' business success	Costly; can hurt more than help if not done well
Gainsharing	Medium	Provides economic benefits for hospital and physicians	Short-lived; takes time to implement
Real estate investment	Medium/high	Opportunity to include primary care physicians	Limited strategic alignment unless building investment tied to strategy
Service line management or comanagement	High	Strong economic and strategic alignment; somewhat easier to unwind if necessary	Contracting potentially complex; requires strong combined vision and agreement on strategic goals and operating principles
Participating bond transactions	High	Strong economic alignment	More difficult to sell/implement

(continued)

Table 3.1. (*continued*)

Strategies	Strength of Economic Alignment	Advantages	Disadvantages
Joint ventures	High	Strong economic and strategic alignment	Costly; challenging to implement and govern; may increase operating costs
Physician employment	High	Strongest alignment; minimizes economic risk for physicians	Significant economic and political risk, especially if incentive compensation is not set up properly
Integrated delivery system/ clinic model	High	Physician-driven organization means high collaboration	High hurdles for implementation; must have significant support from all physicians in a community

Service (IRS) imposed in 1993 for physician membership on the boards of 501(c)(3) tax-exempt healthcare organizations. The rule changed in 1996 to allow up to 49 percent of board membership to be "interested persons." The IRS considers employees and physicians who treat patients of the organization, and who conduct business with or derive any financial benefit from the organization, to be interested persons (Orlikoff and Totten 2005).

Physicians on hospital boards and board committees must be free of material conflicts of interest with the hospital. It is difficult for hospitals, particularly those in smaller communities, to ensure "independence" of physician board members according to IRS guidelines. Hospital boards should develop and implement clear conflict-of-interest policies and procedures; legal review is critical.

MEDICAL DIRECTORSHIPS

A medical directorship involves granting physicians titles and managerial authority over operational and clinical issues in a specific service line or program. Many hospitals use medical directorships to attract physician leaders who can build and sustain strong clinical programs. Hospital leaders must clearly define

the medical directors' duties and outline the hours associated with those duties. Typically, medical directorships are formally established through a contract between the hospital and the physician (or the physician's medical group) or an employment agreement between the two parties.

Compensation, which most often is required to attract key physicians, is specified in the agreement. Some experts recommend that compensation should be based on fair-market standards for the specific duties actually performed and the required number of hours to perform such duties rather than on the opportunity cost of the physician's lost income during such hours (Patel, Khorover, and Pizzo 2007). Benchmarks for medical directorship pay levels are available through associations and commercial sources (see Sidebar 3.4).

The government has increased its scrutiny of medical directorships in view of possible illegal kickback practices, IRS rules prohibiting excessive compensation of key individuals in tax-exempt organizations, and violations of the Stark law, so again, legal counsel is recommended to ensure compliance with relevant laws and regulations.

SIDEBAR 3.3

Physicians on the Board

Average data on board composition for organizations responding to the Governance Institute's most recent survey of hospitals and health systems were as follows:

Board size	13.3 members
Physicians on the medical staff but not employed by the organization	1.8 members
Physicians on the medical staff and employed by the organization	0.4 members
Physicians considered "outside" members (not on staff and not employed)	0.3 members

The chief of staff was a voting member of the board in 42.7 percent of responding hospitals and health systems, a nonvoting board member in 11.2 percent, and a regularly attending nonboard member in 35.8 percent.

Source: The Governance Institute. 2007a. *Boards × 4. Governance Structures and Practices: The 2007 Biennial Survey of Hospitals and Healthcare Systems.* San Diego, CA: The Governance Institute. Used with permission.

SIDEBAR 3.4

Selected Sources for Benchmark Data on Medical Director/ Executive Compensation

- *2007 Physician Executive Compensation Survey* (American College of Physician Executives and Cejka Search 2007) www.cejkasearch.com
- *2007 Medical Director Survey* (Clark Consulting 2007) www.clarkconsulting.com
- *Management Compensation Survey: 2007 Report Based on 2006 Data* (Medical Group Management Association 2007) www.mgma.com

PHYSICIAN SUPPORT STRATEGIES

Hospitals use numerous strategies to provide physician practice support (see Sidebar 3.5). One increasingly common strategy involves *forgivable loans.* These are often used to recruit physicians to work for a hospital or to establish a practice in the hospital's service area. For example, Palomar Pomerado Health, a two-hospital system in San Diego County, is offering legally structured partial-loan forgiveness to young PCPs who are willing to locate in the expensive county, and it is providing hospital-based educational opportunities for University of California, San Diego, residency programs (Grube, Gish, and Tkach 2008).

Malpractice Insurance

Numerous hospitals use malpractice pools as a strategy to offer independent physicians lower malpractice costs, thereby enhancing loyalty and retention. Through self-insurance, hospitals gain direct involvement and influence over the insurance operations, including underwriting and claims management, but they must be able to manage risk and minimize adverse claims. If a self-insured hospital does not properly plan and reserve for losses, the organization's

financial position can be significantly harmed (Brierton 2004). In addition, obtaining affordable reinsurance, which covers losses above a specified level, has become increasingly expensive for self-insured hospitals (Mello 2006).

Technology

Information technology assistance and linkage is a key strategy that

---

SIDEBAR 3.5

Physician Practice Support Strategies

The following data are from a national survey of strategies hospitals use to help strengthen physician-hospital relationships, conducted for the Society for Healthcare Strategy and Market Development. Percentages indicate use of strategy by the 300 responding hospitals.

Strategy	Percent Using Strategy
Financial support for recruitment to independent practices	83%
Training to physician office staff to improve coding, billing, and collections	56%
Information system support for independent practices	53%
A formal physician relations program to grow referrals to the hospital and its physicians	50%
Other types of management support for independent practices (accounting, credentialing, contract negotiations)	46%
Advertise independent physicians (provide marketing support for physicians and actively advertise their practices)	37%

Source: McGowan, R.A. and A.S. MacNulty. 2005. "Strategies for Strengthening Physician-Hospital Alignment: A National Study," Noblis (formerly Mitretek Systems, Inc.), Chicago: Society for Healthcare Marketing and Strategy Development. Used with permission.

should be considered by all hospitals. Providing assistance to physicians in the area of IT can yield significant mutual benefits related to quality of care, care outcomes, and patient satisfaction.

Although most physicians recognize the importance of an EHR system in reducing medication and other errors and enhancing care coordination, many physicians, particularly PCPs, are not able to implement such systems without financial and logistical support and incentives.

The development of a formal technology strategy for EHRs and a formal "online" linkage for results reporting will be critical in the future, particularly to PCPs. Many physicians finishing residencies and considering where to establish practice will be looking for technology to improve or enhance their patient care and lifestyle experience. Hospitals that make the investment in technology and communicate their technology plan will be better able to recruit and retain physicians.

The next five years will be a critical juncture for IT in healthcare. Organizations that are investing in EHRs, electronic prescribing, and other systems that are linked to on-staff and community-based physicians will increasingly be able to achieve quality

outcomes and improve patient safety. The "have-not" hospitals will have a very tough time catching up. According to the credit rating agencies, attention to healthcare IT will enable hospitals to achieve their quality initiatives and will be a differentiating factor in hospital credit quality (Moody's Investors Service 2007; Fitch Ratings 2006).

Hospitals not ready to assume major IT projects should start with a project with a limited scope—for example, emergency department management—and work with the staff and physicians to make the required process changes. A significant proportion of the IT design and implementation "battle" is preparing the organization for change. Smaller, stand-alone facilities might also consider exploring IT partnerships with larger providers and multi-hospital systems. Such partnerships can help smaller organizations gain access to sophisticated IT at less cost than developing their own capacity and allow the larger organizations to leverage their IT investment.

Digital imaging and picture archiving and communication systems are particularly important, as are physician practice management systems. Because hospitals are likely to be employing more physicians in the future, as described later in the chapter, good systems will make a difference in demonstrating quality outcomes and reduced costs.

Centers for Medicare & Medicaid Services and Office of the Inspector General (OIG) rules effective in October 2006 provide that donations of technology to support and promote physician adoption of e-prescribing and EHRs will not violate Stark and antikickback laws. Hospitals can donate hardware, software, and training services to physicians if certain conditions are met, such as requirements related to cost sharing and execution of a written agreement. Legal counsel is advised.

Communication with Generalists and Specialists

To align their interests and enhance physician referrals, hospitals can consider ways to facilitate communication between specialists, PCPs, and the hospital.

For example, Gundersen Lutheran Health System in La Crosse, Wisconsin, has developed an extensive regional referral network program that includes 1,500 physicians and other rural providers (Grube 2007). The organization's detailed and comprehensive provider database and innovative "feedback loop" communication system keeps referring physicians informed about the care their patients receive in the hospital.

A Physician Relations Program

The next example comes from a not-for-profit health system, which owns and operates hospitals, ambulatory health and surgery centers, home health agencies, and medical equipment and health service suppliers throughout a multicounty area in one state. This health system, which has more than 10,000 employees and 2,000 physicians, achieved approximately 100,000 inpatient admissions and more than 300,000 emergency department visits in 2007. More than half of the physicians in the system's market area are affiliated with the health system.

PHYSICIAN RELATIONS CONCEPT. Directed by a senior hospital executive who is responsible for physician relations and development, the system's six-person physician relations staff serves as "the face" of the system with physicians and their office staff. Their focus is on PCPs and specialists as customers, using a service-driven, relationship-based program modeled after the approach used in the pharmaceutical industry. Physicians are identified based on their profile as being "loyal" (80 percent or greater of their admissions to system hospitals) or a "splitter" (less than 80 percent of admissions to system hospitals). The goal is to build and solidify relationships with physicians and office staff through the provision of a consistent level of service and communication.

TOOLS AND TACTICS. Physician office visits, peer interactions, and issue resolution are the primary approaches used by the physician relations staff. The staff visits more than 500 physicians throughout the state every six to eight weeks, with the goal being to present the physicians and their staff with current information regarding selected products and service lines.

The physician relations staff takes new physicians, medical specialists, administrators, and appropriate clinical personnel to referring physicians' offices to facilitate interaction and introductions. This activity often results in strengthening existing or creating new physician relationships.

The goal of issue resolution initiatives is to identify and reduce barriers for physician offices. The program has made a 24–48 hour problem-resolution pledge and monitors resolution efforts through a database system.

For example, one of the key, but splitter, PCPs in the area, with six family practitioners, expressed a sense of disenfranchisement. Issues raised included the system's employment of PCPs in close proximity, the need for IT connectivity with the system, and the desire for the system's general surgeon to time-share with the practice.

In response, the system did the following:

■ Assigned a physician relations representative to visit the office more frequently and facilitated a meeting with the hospital president
■ Provided loan and co-marketing assistance to two system family practice residents who joined the practice
■ Offered access to the system's browser, which gives clinicians and their staff results data from all inpatient and outpatient encounters in area system-affiliated hospitals
■ Provided the opportunity to gain access to the system's EMR
■ Successfully facilitated placement of the general surgeon

HOSPITAL-PHYSICIAN RELATIONS SUPPORT SYSTEM. Operated through an account management system, this initiative aims to enhance relationships with hundreds of specialists who practice at system-affiliated hospitals through quarterly visits by executives and issue resolution within 14 days.

Other Strategies

Hospitals with many affiliated solo or small-group physicians in private practice may also wish to consider developing a primary care network that offers physician-to-physician and physician-to-hospital assistance with contracting, IT, and/or quality improvement initiatives.

Many hospitals provide marketing and business development assistance to PCPs. This may be an effective means to help physicians grow their practices. MemorialCare Medical Centers and Palomar Pomerado Health, both located in competitive geographic areas in California, are opening "minute clinics," whose hospital name-branding capabilities in the market are central to the strategy of increasing referrals to PCPs and the hospital.

Palomar Pomerado Health also recently secured a 20-year agreement with wellness-focused managed-care giant Kaiser Permanente, which allows Kaiser physicians to use Palomar Pomerado Health facilities (Grube, Gish, and Tkach 2008).

Offering physicians convenient office space in a building near or attached to a hospital can also build loyalty and referrals. Unlike alignment opportunities with specialists/proceduralists, the options (financial or otherwise) to engage PCPs with the hospital are more limited, so creativity may be needed (see Figure 3.2).

PHYSICIAN-HOSPITAL ORGANIZATIONS

A PHO is a legal entity formed by a hospital and one or more physicians or physician groups for the purpose of negotiating and obtaining contracts with insurance plans and employers. Physicians maintain ownership of their practices and often significant business outside the PHO, but they agree to accept managed care patients according to the terms of a professional services agreement with the PHO. Physician-hospital organizations originated during the 1980s with the rise of managed care and were widely prevalent by the mid-1990s.

The PHO typically is owned and governed jointly by a hospital and shareholder physicians. It may provide various services to its members, such as utilization review, credential-

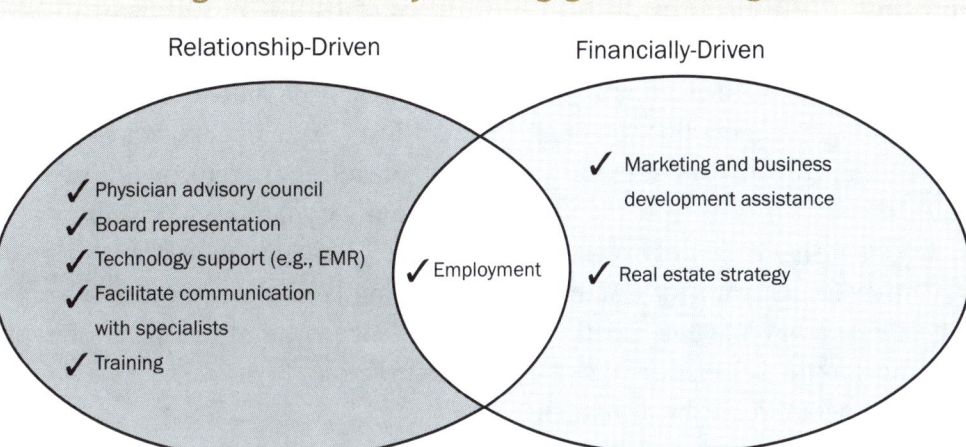

Figure 3.2. Primary Care Engagement Strategies

Relationship-Driven   Financially-Driven

✓ Physician advisory council
✓ Board representation
✓ Technology support (e.g., EMR)
✓ Facilitate communication
  with specialists
✓ Training

✓ Employment

✓ Marketing and business
  development assistance

✓ Real estate strategy

Source: Kaufman, Hall & Associates, Inc. Used with permission.

ing, and quality assurance. Physician-hospital organizations provide some economic alignment between hospitals and physicians, but physician loyalty may be to the contracts, not the hospital. The advantages include leverage with payers, low capital investment requirements, and potentially a new stream of patients for hospitals and physicians.

On the negative side, there is no guarantee that payment will increase through PHOs, and economies of scale with payer negotiations may require including physicians that do not perform well. Many PHOs have failed, for reasons including the inability of the independent groups to agree on contract terms or to secure

rates that exceed what the independent groups could do on their own. The complexity of PHO management has proven challenging to many PHO participants.

CENTERS OF EXCELLENCE OR CLINICAL INSTITUTES

Centers of excellence are state-of-the-art clinical programs or institutes, generally operated within a hospital, for which top specialists are recruited and which are recognized for the provision of sophisticated service offerings and high-quality care in the relevant specialty(ies). These "virtual entities" are designed to integrate the strategic, high-profile clinical goals of the hospital or health system with those of a group of specialty physicians around such efforts as establishing a market-differentiating standard of care and services for patients.

To establish a center of excellence in cardiovascular care, for example, a hospital would integrate existing programs in the selected service line, extend program reach by developing physician referral relationships and program-specific marketing initiatives, recruit additional physicians, establish a dedicated inpatient space and resources (nursing teams, surgical teams), and reinforce the program with disease management and wellness promotion.

The goal for hospitals is to achieve increased volume, improved clinical outcomes and patient satisfaction, and cost efficiencies. Physicians associated with a center of excellence should achieve increased patient satisfaction and practice efficiencies. Centers of excellence or clinical institutes do not align hospitals and physicians economically unless combined with another strategy, such as joint venture ownership or comanagement arrangements, as described later.

The success of this strategy has been highly variable. The organiza-

tions that have succeeded are those that make a serious resource investment in the programs and those that have been able to attract strong physician leaders. Less successful organizations are typically those without a dynamic and visionary physician champion and/or those that simply market their centers of excellence without really investing in the program.

MANAGEMENT SERVICES ORGANIZATIONS

A management services organization (MSO) is an organization wholly owned by a hospital or health system or jointly owned with physicians, whose function is to provide administrative, practice management, and/or asset management services to physicians and physician groups. Management services organizations provide services in exchange for either a flat fee or a defined percentage of group revenues.

Management services organizations are typically a direct subsidiary of a hospital, but they may be owned by investors, including physicians. Management services organizations that are established as limited liability companies (LLCs), representing a joint venture between a hospital and physician group, provide revenue to physician owners when the MSO is profitable, thereby improving economic alignment. Hospitals may be particularly interested in MSOs because the arrangement offers a way to support and improve the financial performance of physician practices without having to acquire the practice or employ the physicians. Through offering such benefits as malpractice insurance through insurance pools and IT infrastructure that enables physicians to access EHRs, MSOs can significantly reduce physicians' overhead costs. Physicians who do not wish to be employed by hospitals may find this an attractive collaborative alternative.

Management services organizations require intensive physician practice management skills, which healthcare executives have started to gain in the past decade, as well as the effective balancing of day-to-day practice operations and long-term strategic decisions. Some MSOs have gained this competency through contracts with national physician practice management companies that have well-established and deep experience in physician practice management.

While intuitively appealing, the success rate for MSOs, like PHOs, has been less than compelling. Successful physician practice managers need to manage costs at a micro level, which is inconsistent with managerial practices at many hospitals. The inability to attract a large pool of physicians to the MSO also limits economies of scale, which, in turn, limits efficiency gains. Additionally, if not carefully implemented, shifting to new and different managerial protocols can result in decreased physician and patient satisfaction.

GAINSHARING

Gainsharing involves a contractual arrangement between a hospital and physician group(s) in which the hospital agrees to pay the physicians a share of the cost savings related to specific cost-reduction initiatives. The goal is to encourage the implementation of such initiatives through economic alignment of the parties.

Gainsharing contracts have typically been used in high-cost areas for hospitals, such as cardiac services. In such areas, specific practice changes, such as standardization of device usage—for example, implantable defibrillators—can significantly reduce operating room and supply costs. No capital investment, beyond that related to obtaining regulatory approval, is required by either party. Economic benefits accrue to both parties.

The OIG has provided narrowly defined guidelines for gainsharing. At this point, approved gainsharing programs are written for a period of one year only, after which they have to be rewritten based on current performance standards. Notes one legal expert, "Because of the amount of time it may take to obtain regulatory approval, many hospitals are choosing to pursue other ventures that are quicker to structure and implement and that have less regulatory risk" (Patel, Khorover, and Pizzo 2007).

REAL ESTATE INVESTMENT

Real estate investment is an increasingly prevalent collaboration strategy. Using this strategy, a hospital offers physicians a percentage of ownership in, for example, a new medical office building in which the hospital is investing. Real estate investment can involve many types of properties, from physician office buildings to the land on which ambulatory centers are built.

Under the equity participation model, a single-purpose LLC or a limited partnership is formed to own or ground lease the real estate. Funds required for development can be obtained from the hospital or health system, a real estate organization, qualified physicians and physician group investors, and construction loan proceeds. Physicians generally make passive financial investments, are not responsible for property ownership, and may have the right to lease space in the property (Davis 2007).

Under the interest model, the real estate is held by a real estate organization, which funds the development and incurs all risk. The hospital or health system and physicians/physician groups make lease commitments for the associated property. The real estate organization offers the participants with lease commitments a percentage interest in the profit, depending on the amount of space leased. Participants are not required to make any equity contributions, but the total maximum percentage of profits paid to participants is capped at a defined percentage (for example, 40 percent). Prior to making profit payments, the real estate organization is entitled to a minimum internal rate of return on its invested funds and to market-based fees for services provided.

Hospitals should ensure that they develop a real estate deal for the right strategic reasons and not simply for the sake of aligning with physicians. If real estate makes sense for the organization, the organization can offer physicians an interest. Although an inclusive approach is recommended, considerations include whether to offer investment opportunities to private practice and employed physicians and the size of the investment required of physicians. Offering small investment increments can attract physicians who want a "piece of the action," but do not have a lot of capital.

SERVICE LINE MANAGEMENT OR COMANAGEMENT

This strategy involves a contractual agreement between a hospital and a management services company, which is formed by a group of physicians. Through this company, the physician group agrees to perform clinical and operational management services for a defined hospital service line (see Figure 3.3). The hospital retains the license and billing and collection services and pays the management company on a fixed-fee or per-case basis. Typically, performance incentives are also built into the contracts.

This strategy, often called "co-management," allows physicians to invest in a company whose goal is to improve operations at the hospital where they have admitting privileges. Quality and efficiency improvements achieved through operational efficiency and patient care standards will benefit the hospital and physicians, but broad participation of physicians in the specialty is

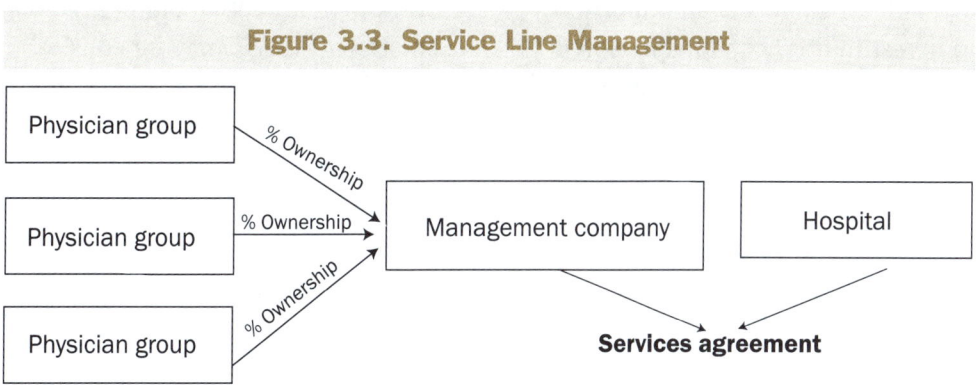

Figure 3.3. Service Line Management

Source: Kaufman, Hall & Associates, Inc. Used with permission.

required. If the busiest and highest-revenue–producing physicians do not participate, success will be limited. The hospital has to be willing to give up a certain amount of control related to strategy and clinical operations. This involves risk for hospitals, so hospitals must have a high degree of confidence in the participating physicians.

Sidebar 3.6 provides critical success factors offered by the executive of a health system that has established a number of successful comanagement agreements.

PARTICIPATING BOND TRANSACTIONS

Participating bond transactions (PBTs) are an alternative to equity joint ventures for not-for-profit hospitals. Typically sold as subordinated instruments, PBTs enable hospitals to offer their physicians an opportunity to invest in the hospital-sponsored taxable or tax-free municipal bonds, typically at a higher-than-usual rate of return.

Participating bond transactions can be used to create an investment opportunity in any facility that could be structured as a joint venture, such as an ambulatory surgery center or imaging center, and can also be used

with existing and replacement facilities (Rosenfield 2005). The amount of interest investors earn on these bonds is based on the economic performance of the entity on behalf of which the bonds have been issued. Bond performance can also be linked to other nonfinancial indicators, such as improvement in quality of patient care or patient satisfaction.

Although not yet a commonly used strategy, PBTs may be considered by hospitals with strong credit ratings and solid balance sheets. They generally are expensive in terms of the cost of the capital and the legal fees, but, when used to finance projects of strategic importance to physicians, they can be very effective in creating a strong financial tie between the hospital and participating physicians. Physicians bear very little risk but can achieve solid returns.

JOINT VENTURES

For the purposes of this book, a joint venture is any short- or long-term arrangement involving risk and benefit sharing between a hospital or health system and one or more physician groups or individual physicians to form and operate a common enterprise.

Clinical service delivery is the core purpose of many joint ventures, including ambulatory surgery centers, imaging facilities, endoscopy centers, urgent care centers, oncology centers, outpatient diagnostic and treatment facilities, and specialty hospitals. Hospitals are also entering into joint ventures with physicians and other partners to own and operate MSOs, medical office buildings, and other entities.

Whether pursued proactively, re-actively, or by a combination thereof, joint ventures with physicians represent a strategy that can be especially helpful in strengthening relationships with physicians and aligning economic incentives to enhance market position and ultimately financial success. Joint ventures can offer high

financial rewards for physicians and enable hospitals to expand inpatient and outpatient capacity at a shared cost, while stemming the competition between the parties. Joint ventures often, however, involve loss of technical revenue for hospitals; but as many point out, "50 percent of something is better than 100 percent of nothing." In highly competitive markets, joint ventures with physicians may, in fact, be the most (or only) viable way for hospitals to ensure that they are not competing head-to-head with physicians. This can have a significant effect on a hospital's clinical programs beyond the joint venture. As one rating agency notes, "As more and more profitable services are removed from the hospital into joint ventures, the organization impairs its ability to cost shift from less profitable, but essential, clinical services" (Fitch Ratings 2007).

Joint venture policy development is too often overlooked by healthcare organizations. As a result, management teams and governing boards lack the benefit of a broader context within which to evaluate specific opportunities brought forward by physicians and other for-profit or not-for-profit entities. The context defines where the venture fits within the organization's strategic, financial, and operating plans and the terms under which the organization is willing to enter into a joint relationship.

Questions to determine policies and principles for joint venture involvement include the following:

- Are we interested only in ventures that are somehow connected to the mission and vision of the organization?
- Are we willing to enter a venture in which we hold a minority position?
- Do we establish a principle of proportionality related to investment in equity/ownership of the joint venture? If so, what should it be?
- Are we willing to establish a joint venture with a subset of medical staff physicians in a particular specialty?
- Are we willing to operate a venture as a truly separate entity?
- How much risk are we willing to take related to potential regulatory challenges?
- Have the parameters of the "unwind" of the venture been established and are they consistent with our policies and principals?

Development of a policy document that includes the elements out-

SIDEBAR 3.7

Components of a Joint Venture Policy

- Statement of purpose
- Definitions
- Guidelines for joint venture review, evaluation, approval, and management
  - Legal guidance/participation requirements
  - Screening and approval process (with process diagram)
    - Initial proposal approval request (guidelines and form)
    - Development of business plan (guidelines and review form)
    - Required financial analytics
    - Approval process
  - Management and operating guidelines
    - Reporting and self-assessment requirements
- Divestiture or withdrawal process

Source: Blaszyk, M. D., and J. Hill-Mischell. 2007. *Joint Ventures: From Policy to Post-Execution Monitoring.* Skokie, IL: Kaufman, Hall & Associates, Inc. Used with permission.

lined in Sidebar 3.7 can be helpful in guiding assessment and decision making.

Structure and governance of joint ventures are key issues (see Sidebar 3.8). In equity joint ventures, services are provided by a new legal entity that is owned by physicians, the hospital, and potentially a third party, typically as an LLC or limited partnership. The new entity has its own tax identification number, separate from the hospital or physicians, and contracts separately with commercial payers (see Figure 3.4). In many instances, the hospital and/or a third party provides the capital, and expenses and revenues are interest when the physician investors bring more than the hospital to the joint venture table. The risk assumed by joint venture partners is directly proportional to their equity and governance position.

The final Stark III rule, released by CMS in September 2007, prohibits or significantly scrutinizes specific types of physician-hospital joint ventures, so many hospitals have unwound or are currently unwinding or restructuring such ventures.

Physician-hospital joint ventures are extremely complex arrangements, and, because they involve ongoing relationships, their execution typically is even more complicated than a merger or acquisition. The legal requirements related to structure and financing are intricate, so expert advice is mandatory.

EMPLOYMENT

Hospitals traditionally have employed or entered into employment-like contractual arrangements with physicians in hospital-based specialties, such as radiology, anesthesiology, and emergency medicine, but a much broader range of employment is now under way. Hospitals not already employing specialty and PCPs should be prepared to do so.

shared by the three parties according to predetermined percentages.

Percentage of ownership is one of the most significant issues addressed in joint venture structuring. Some hospitals insist on a 51 percent ownership; others are more willing to consider less than a majority

Figure 3.4. Equity Joint Venture Model

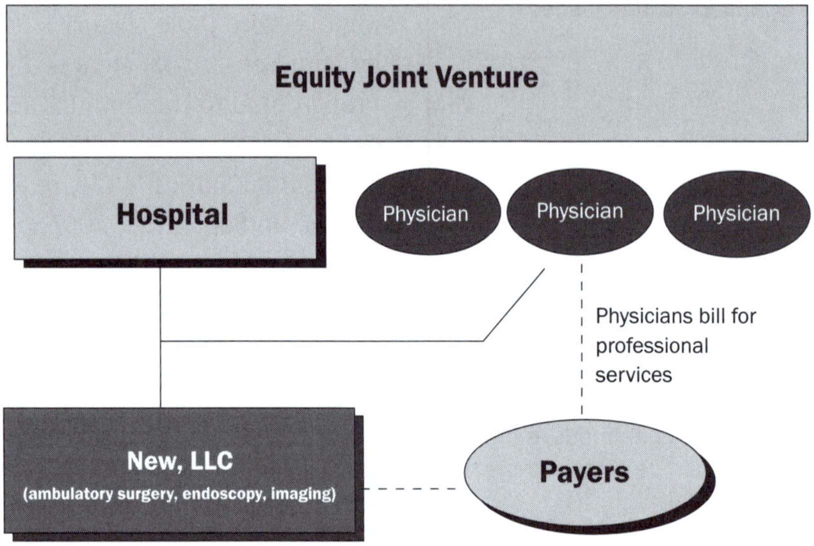

Source: Reprinted from Cohen, R. L., undated. "Physician-Hospital Joint Venture and Affiliation Models." Omaha, NE: Kutak Rock. Used with permission.

To ensure survival of primary care practices and retain referrals, employment of PCPs is again at the forefront of hospitals' physician initiatives. Current hospital success in owning physician practices and employing physicians is generally better than in the previous decade (see Sidebar 3.9).

Employment of specialists in hard-to-recruit fields is also on the rise to ensure provision of needed services in the market. "Our real issue is not *if* we are going to employ physicians, but *how* we are going to employ them," says one CEO of a hospital that employs PCPs and specialists. "Located in a rural area and with payments as low as they are, physicians just can't afford to be in practice or recruit to their practice the

---

SIDEBAR 3.9

Ownership of Physician Practices: Then and Now

In the 1990s
- Ineffective management
- Declining fee-for-service payment
- Poor revenue-cycle performance
- Decreased productivity
- Increased overhead
- Significant goodwill payments

In the 2000s
- Improved management
- Benefits of IT
- Quality and cost reduction initiatives
- Productivity/revenue-based compensation
- Payment for hard assets only

colleagues they need" (The Governance Institute 2007b).

The importance of a demonstrated track record of effective physician engagement, recruitment, and retention cannot be underestimated. Physicians will join and stay when hospitals:

- align organizational and physician economic interests;
- seek physician input to and participation with decision making that affects clinical service lines; and
- provide a positive, collaborative organizational culture with the facilities, clinical support staff, and technology needed to ensure high-quality patient care and patient satisfaction.

Effective compensation plans will be critical to recruiting and retaining the best physicians. Laws in some states, such as California, Texas, Ohio, Colorado, and others, prohibit hospital employment of physi-

cians for the provision of outpatient services, so legal counsel should be obtained early. In these situations, alternatives may be available (e.g., a foundation model) that can accomplish the desired objective under a different organizational structure(s).

Models for employment vary widely. Their description is beyond this book's scope but available from professional associations and commercial sources. Non–hospital-based employed physicians generally work for a separate, nonobligated corporation. Tax laws are complex and can affect hospital financial performance.

The best compensation plans for physicians, whether based on salary, salary plus bonus, productivity, or a combination thereof, consider additional issues, such as strategic contribution, patient satisfaction, governance and leadership, teamwork, panel size, pay-for-performance clinical data outcomes, medical loss ratio, benchmarks, and performance monitoring. Solid data are required to effectively monitor performance with each compensation component. Revenue generated, salaries, and productivity by specialty are highly relevant, widely varied, and constantly changing. Data are readily available through numerous sources (see Sidebar 3.10).

SIDEBAR 3.10

A Sampling of Physician Salary, Productivity, and Revenue Data Sources
- American College of Physician Executives (www.acpe.org)
- American Medical Group Association (www.amga.org)
- Medical Group Management Association (www.mgma.org)
- Merritt Hawkins & Associates (www.merritthawkins.com)
- Sullivan, Cotter and Associates (www.sullivancotter.com)

Figure 3.5. Average Hospital Revenue (Inpatient and Outpatient) Generated by Physician Specialty

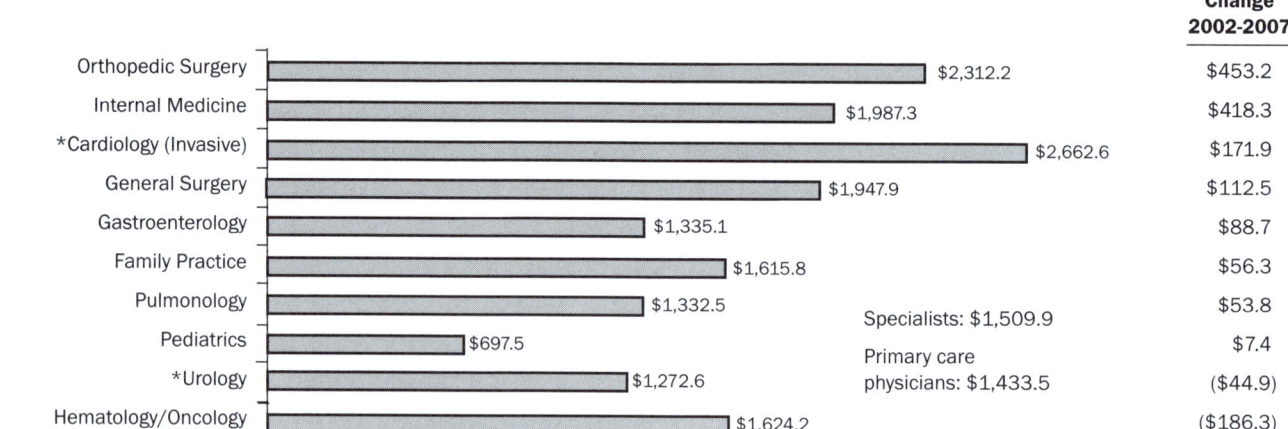

Specialty	Revenue ($000s)	Change 2002-2007
Orthopedic Surgery	$2,312.2	$453.2
Internal Medicine	$1,987.3	$418.3
*Cardiology (Invasive)	$2,662.6	$171.9
General Surgery	$1,947.9	$112.5
Gastroenterology	$1,335.1	$88.7
Family Practice	$1,615.8	$56.3
Pulmonology	$1,332.5	$53.8
Pediatrics	$697.5	$7.4
*Urology	$1,272.6	($44.9)
Hematology/Oncology	$1,624.2	($186.3)
Obstetrics/Gynecology	1,413.4	($229.6)
Psychiatry	$888.9	($249.1)
Neurosurgery	$2,100.0	($264.9)
Neurology	$557.9	($472.4)
*Cardiology (Noninvasive)	$2,240.8	($405.3)
Nephrology	$865.2	($839.1)
Ophthalmology	$584.3	NA

Specialists: $1,509.9

Primary care physicians: $1,433.5

* Shows change between 2004 and 2007; data for 2002 not available.

Source: Adapted with permission from Merritt, Hawkins & Associates. 2007. "2007 Physician Inpatient/Outpatient Revenue Survey." [Online information; retrieved 3/08.] http://merritthawkins.com/pdf2007_Physician_Inpatient_Outpatient_Revenue_Survey.pdf.

Some would advise that compensation plans are so volatile that there really only are three pay plans—last year's, this year's, and next year's. A structure to establish and monitor how salary decisions are made can reduce volatility and separate subjectivity from objectivity.

Figure 3.5 indicates average annual hospital revenue by specialty and how such revenue changed during a recent five-year period. Figure 3.6 shows the relationship of average hospital revenue by specialty to starting salaries in the specialty. Internists and family practitioners

Figure 3.6. Average Revenue Generated vs. Average Starting Salary by Physician Specialty

Specialty	Hospital Inpatient/ Outpatient Revenue ($000s)	Average Starting Physician Salary ($000s)	Revenue-to-Salary Ratio
Internal Medicine	1,987.3	162.0	12.3
Family Practice	1,615.8	145.0	11.1
Cardiology (invasive)	2,662.6	342.0	7.8
General Surgery	1,947.9	272.0	7.2
Cardiology (noninvasive)	2,240.3	342.0	6.6
Orthopedic Surgery	2,312.2	370.0	6.2
Obstetrics/Gynecology	1,413.4	234.0	6.0
Hematology/Oncology	1,624.2	275.0	5.9
Pulmonology	1,332.5	248.0	5.4
Psychiatry	888.9	174.0	5.1
Pediatrics	697.5	151.0	4.6
Neurosurgery	2,100.0	489.0	4.3
Gastroenterology	1,336.1	315.0	4.2
Urology	1,272.6	320.0	4.0
Nephrology	865.2	225.0	3.8
Neurology	557.9	210.0	2.7
Ophthalmology	584.3	N/A	N/A

Source: Adapted with permission from Merritt, Hawkins & Associates. 2007. "2007 Physician Inpatient/Outpatient Revenue Survey." [Online information; retrieved 3/08.] http://merritt hawkins.com/pdf2007_Physician_Inpatient_Outpatient_Revenue_Survey.pdf.

generate revenue of approximately 11 to 12 times their starting salary; the specialists with the highest starting salaries (neurosurgery and orthopedic surgery) generate annual revenues of approximately 4 to 6 times their starting salaries. Data such as these are helpful to hospitals in shaping expectations and compensation plans.

Challenges for hospitals in employing physicians include the complexities associated with compensation, quality initiatives, and cost. In addition, hospitals must address the concerns of independent medical staff about direct competition from the hospital's employed physicians. Employment of some physicians can alienate others, so an effective balancing of employed and on-staff physicians is critical.

INTEGRATED DELIVERY SYSTEM/CLINIC MODEL

An integrated delivery system (IDS)/ clinic model is a full-service or multi-specialty organization that employs its physicians and whose focus is generally on integration and coordination of care among all levels and types of care across the continuum. The organization may have begun as a physician group practice, such as what occurred with Cleveland Clinic, or it may have evolved through reorganization of a hospital or health system into a physician-led clinic organization, representing a new legal entity, such as what is occurring with Carilion Clinic (see later example).

Advantages of this model of engagement for physicians include increased input and authority over patient care and hospital and ancillary service operations. Physicians experience income stability through employment, protection from costs associated with private practice,

and lifestyle improvements through shared call coverage. Advantages for the parent organization include revenue stability in competitive markets, a better vehicle for recruitment of physicians, growth through practice capitalization, and the ability to gain the active participation and support of physicians in quality and cost-management efforts. Most important, parent organizations benefit from the accountability physicians then have for all aspects of clinical, operational, and financial outcomes. A report from a credit rating agency notes that a physician-led clinic model might improve the organization's ability to hire renowned physicians in key specialties and increase attention on education and research (Standard & Poor's 2007).

Establishing the model can be very expensive and take substantial energy and time (multiple years). Management and physicians must be committed to organizational change and be able to address the potentially substantial physician resistance in the early stages from community physicians not interested in being employed by the IDS or clinic or preferring an autonomous practice over the integration and coordination of care expected in a clinic.

Example: From Health System to Clinic

In June 2006, Carilion Health System in southwest Virginia commenced the process of becoming "Carilion Clinic," thereby changing from a multihospital health system with independent, affiliated physicians to a physician-led IDS with fully employed physicians (Andrews 2007).

The change reflected the organization's belief that a clinic model, like that used by Cleveland Clinic, would be the best way to address issues, including the following:

- *Quality*: Access issues and physician shortages created by an aging medical staff; inability of private physician groups to recruit and retain physicians; issues with call coverage; the need for closer alignment to drive performance improvement initiatives; and the need for a patient focus in care coordination. Physicians traditionally provided care in a fragmented and inefficient manner with inadequate accountability for outcomes.
- *Financial*: Located in a slow-growth market area, the health system could not achieve organic growth and experienced rising costs and limited opportunity for further cost-reduction initiatives.

Physicians were not properly aligned financially; their accountability for reducing variation in care and consistently applying evidence-based care to reduce care costs and improve value for the community was inadequate.

The transformation involved a new governance structure with a physician-controlled clinical board that has clinical and administrative decision-making powers. The parent company and community-based board remained unchanged but took the new name of Carilion Clinic. The new Carilion Clinic board of governors, with 11 members (CEO, CFO, COO, chief medical officer, chief nursing officer, six physicians with rotating terms, and other executive vice presidents as nonmember staff) manages the entire system, not just the physicians, and assumes responsibility for coordinating all care and activities.

Physicians are employed through Carilion Medical Center, where the flagship hospital is located, and the Carilion Medical Group, a large group of PCPs purchased by the organization. All physicians are organized and led through a departmental structure, which is designed to promote integration, coordination of care, teamwork, and shared accountability for results.

The physician compensation model aims to provide equitable compensation with incentives for alignment. The salary target is set at 10 percent below national benchmarks, with a productivity bonus provided on top of the salary. This bonus is based on a productivity target set at 10 percent below expected productivity and offers the potential of up to 20 percent of salary. Base salaries are determined based on fair pay for the effort required and by ensuring congruence between salary level and productivity expectations (i.e., median base with median productivity; higher bases with higher productivity). A scorecard bonus for quality, efficiency, access, service,

performance in education and research programs, and citizenship performance also adds the potential for 20 percent of salary. The total compensation is adjusted based on the physician's interest and type of work—for example, physicians interested in medical research, education, or management would have different salary/productivity/scorecard targets.

CONCLUDING COMMENTS

Chapter 3 has outlined key physician-hospital engagement options; the next and final chapter addresses a best-practice process for selecting and implementing the options deemed most likely to meet the hospital's strategic objectives.

CHAPTER 4

How Do We Develop a Successful Strategy?

Successful physician-hospital engagement strategies are developed within the framework of the organization's overall integrated strategic financial plan. A high-quality, integrated plan seeks to maximize outcomes while reducing risk of failure and generating a profitable bottom line that ensures ongoing competitive performance through strong capital reinvestment. Strategies to align interests with physicians are critical components of this plan, as described earlier.

The planning process begins with the structured assessment outlined in Chapter 2. This assessment provides hospital leadership with a comprehensive understanding of physicians' perceptions of the hospital and general state of mind about future practice plans, opportunities, and challenges. Interviews of physicians conducted by neutral ▶

third parties offer a relatively easy way to gain physician perspectives on perceived quality and availability of care, areas for improvement related to physician-hospital relationships, and recommendations for future hospital engagement with physicians.

But these steps are not enough. A number of key cultural sensitivities, process considerations, organizational factors, and specific leadership competencies and practices, as outlined in Sidebar 4.1, contribute to success in initiatives with physicians. This chapter focuses on selected issues that are resolved through a formal collaboration structure.

BUILDING A COLLABORATIVE CULTURE AND STRUCTURE

Much has been written about the difference in "culture" between physicians and hospital executives, with physicians described as fiercely independent doers who value autonomy, and hospital executives described as planners who work in teams through meetings. Stereotypes diffuse when hospitals and physicians seek and achieve common ground. The provision of high-quality care

---

SIDEBAR 4.1

The Road Map for Successful Physician Initiatives

1. Understand the current situation, including general and specific organizational and physician cultural characteristics that could affect the success of physician initiatives.
2. Define organization's mission and vision and its goals specific to physician strategy.
3. Define success metrics (financial, quality, market share, satisfaction, etc.).
4. Prepare leadership for success by providing education regarding legal considerations, engagement options, and financial considerations.
5. Structure the organization for success in terms of governance, physician leadership, medical staff support infrastructure, medical staff development and recruiting, physician relations, research and education support, and IT.
6. Develop the right strategies (overall physician strategy related to employment, primary care, and specialties, and service-line specific strategy considerations, such as trends and technology), anticipate competitor response, and develop a scenario plan.
7. Measure success and improve by using key metrics with real-time monitoring/planning in a consistent, periodic process.

Source: Kaufman, Hall & Associates, Inc. Used with permission.

---

through effective teamwork between physicians and hospital-based staff, including nurses, pharmacists, and technicians, is a common attribute of "high-functioning hospitals" that achieve a culture of collaboration (Wachter 2004).

Trust is the prerequisite for collaboration. Hospitals that have established a culture of trust between administrators and physicians will find it easier to develop new initiatives with physicians without heavy reliance on economic incentives;

hospitals that do not have a culture of trust will need to turn to economic incentives to attract and retain physician participation.

Hospital and health system executives also need to understand the unique cultural characteristics of their physician staff and the individuals and physician groups with which they wish to engage. Such understanding ensures the selection of viable engagement strategies. For example, if a hospital wishes to align with a group of orthopedic surgeons that is fiercely independent and highly entrepreneurial, employment is likely to be a completely nonviable option. However, an engagement strategy built around an ambulatory surgery or imaging joint venture might be very successful. Conversely, a group of family practice physicians struggling to make ends meet would not likely be joint venture partner candidates, as the physicians lack the resources to make a meaningful investment. The group may be more interested in engagement through practice management services or employment. A one-size-fits-all strategy rarely works when it comes to physician engagement.

Engaging physicians in strategic decision making often provides a starting point. This sounds obvious, but numerous hospitals lack formal or even informal means to gain physician input and perspective about organizational direction. Without this input, strategic plans are much less likely to be on target or achievable.

Communication must extend beyond operational issues to strategic topics, such as new opportunities and potential competition. Physicians can often provide early information about competitive issues, such as breakthrough procedures/technologies or for-profit companies interested in establishing local ambulatory facilities. By engaging physicians early, hospital leaders ensure the broadest possible radar sweep for competitive threats and ensure the development of growth opportunities most likely to align hospital and physician interests. Physicians look to hospitals with which they are affiliated to develop and implement the long-term collaborative vision and gain physician buy-in. They also expect the hospital to collaboratively develop a formal, market-driven strategy for each service line and communicate that strategy to relevant physician stakeholders. Physicians will not drive these processes—the hospital must do so. Regular interaction between hospital leadership and physicians and physician participation on the board are critical.

A physician (or medical) advisory council provides an excellent means for hospital leaders to involve physicians in strategic decision making (Figure 4.1). It also provides a venue, beyond the formal, legal governance structure, for regular and coordinated communication between the hospital and other physicians.

The first steps toward establishing such a council are to identify council cochairs to develop the council's formal charter, which generally addresses broad goals related to the improvement of care in the service area. The cochairs are responsible for shaping and inviting the desired group of physicians from a cross-section of specialties. The council should also include one representative from hospital administration, who ensures administrative follow-up on action items between meetings and reports relevant activities to both the council and management. Transparency and follow through are vital. A dedicated physician relations staff member can assist in this regard.

Council agenda topics address physician-hospital collaboration, growth opportunities, technology investments, facility planning, and

long-term quality initiatives. The council should meet monthly or more often if possible at the beginning; the hospital should pay physicians a nominal amount for attendance.

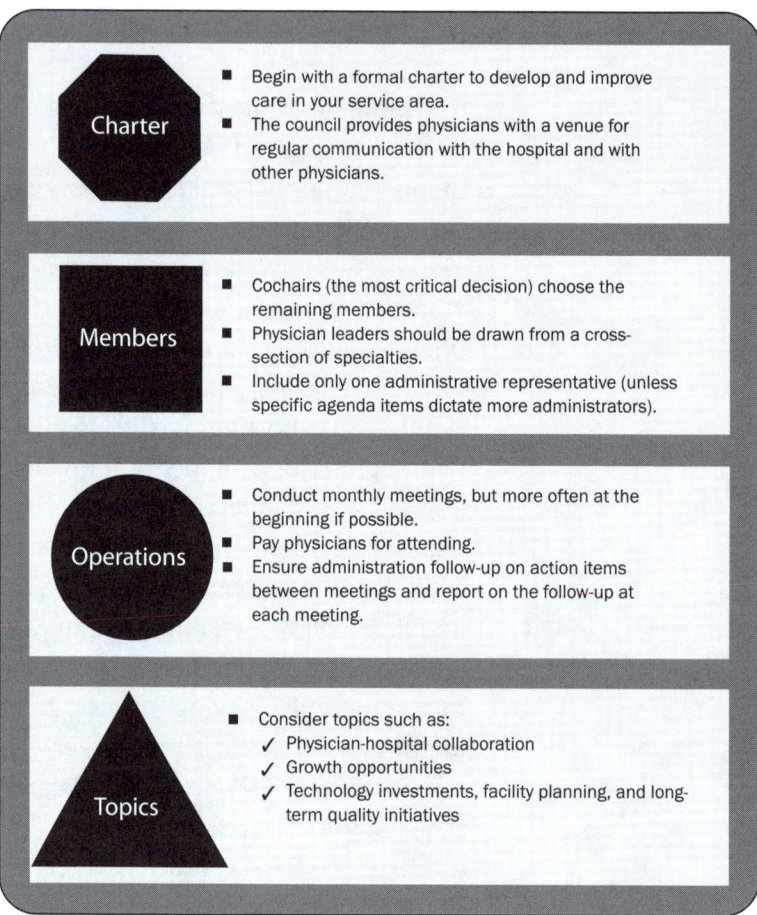

Figure 4.1. Anatomy of a Physician Advisory Council

Charter
- Begin with a formal charter to develop and improve care in your service area.
- The council provides physicians with a venue for regular communication with the hospital and with other physicians.

Members
- Cochairs (the most critical decision) choose the remaining members.
- Physician leaders should be drawn from a cross-section of specialties.
- Include only one administrative representative (unless specific agenda items dictate more administrators).

Operations
- Conduct monthly meetings, but more often at the beginning if possible.
- Pay physicians for attending.
- Ensure administration follow-up on action items between meetings and report on the follow-up at each meeting.

Topics
- Consider topics such as:
  - ✓ Physician-hospital collaboration
  - ✓ Growth opportunities
  - ✓ Technology investments, facility planning, and long-term quality initiatives

Source: Kaufman, Hall & Associates, Inc. Used with permission.

Example: Medical Advisory Panel—A Model for Collaboration

Prior to the development of a medical advisory panel (MAP) at Cottage Health System in California, physician-hospital communication at this three-hospital system was problematic (example drawn from Allyn, Werft, and Warden 2008; Cohn, Allyn, and Reid, 2006). Although a few isolated channels of good communication did exist, there was no organized way for physicians to communicate with administration or the board beyond the medical executive committee, and there was no forum in which physicians could raise new ideas or provide information about program or service-line opportunities.

Based on effective advocacy by the director of medical affairs, Robert A. Reid, MD, who had learned about the MAP concept, the system's board of directors approved formation of such a panel as the forum for structured communication and consideration of strategic priorities. The MAP would report directly to the board and have broad responsibilities. Cottage Health's CEO selected the panel's cochairs, and the cochairs selected 15 members, which included a mix of physicians and surgeons; specialists and generalists; and private practice, clinic-based, and hospital-based physicians. Thomas R. Allyn, MD, Cottage Health's chief of nephrology and cochair of the MAP, says he got "roped into participating" because he was "hospital-phobic" and "administration adverse." "I thought hospitals couldn't change because they were too slow, cumbersome, reticent, consensus-driven, and bureaucratic, but I was wrong. I went to meetings because I was impressed by the quality of my fellow panel members and trusted the commitment made by the board and CEO to give serious consideration to the implementation of the panel's recommendations," said Allyn (Allyn, Werft, and Warden 2008).

The formal goal of the MAP was to evaluate and recommend clinical priorities for the hospital system for the forthcoming three to five years. Consultants facilitated initial meetings of the panel to allow members time to learn how to effectively communicate with each other and to develop, understand, and agree on the collaboration process.

During the first six months, all major clinical service lines and departments provided the panel with detailed information and analyses of their areas' future challenges, opportunities, and needs. The panel also challenged presenters to answer three big-picture questions: Where do we need to be in three to five years? What do we need to do to get there? How will we best accomplish such change? They asked for recommendations that would likely achieve the following: improve clinical outcomes, improve services to patients, fill service voids in the community, strengthen other clinical services, improve physician-to-physician communication, improve hospital and office practice, increase market share, and be cost-effective.

The hospital CEO, directors of nursing and finance, and chief information officer also presented to the panel. Administration provided financial information, with the CFO attending eight meetings in the first year to provide MAP members with tools to understand the financial detail. All presentations and discussions were strictly confidential.

Using a scoring system and tool developed by the consultant, the MAP scored each presentation and reached consensus findings and recommendations of clinical priorities, which the panel reported to the board. The panel also outlined "quick fixes," which were implemented rapidly, adding credibility to the process early. This illustrated to the hospital and physician community that MAP would have an impact on getting physician concerns addressed by administration.

Top program priorities identified by MAP were neurosciences, surgical services, emergency services, palliative care, psychiatric services, and an eye center. One of the panel members, an orthopedist, led his department to a consensus on limiting multiple vendors for joint implants, resulting in a $1.4 million savings in 2004 and continued savings thereafter. The panel's effort to limit sepsis mortality reduced it from the national rate of 46 percent in 2004 to 19 percent in 2006. This rate has been sustained since. "Gains in sepsis mortality reduction were the result of streamlining laboratory and x-ray turnarounds, but most importantly, we were able to accelerate antibiotic administration by dramatically decreasing the time from written order to administration," comments Allyn (2008). Continuing to this day, all major recommendations from the panel have been accepted and implemented by the board of directors or administration.

The benefits of the MAP to Cottage Health System included the following: panel members became "owners" as they developed detailed understanding of hospital decisions; physicians saw they could make a difference and have their voices heard; physicians gained new respect for the complexity of the administration's challenges; administration could embark on new programs and ventures with full support of the medical staff and board approval; and the active engagement of the medical staff through this process strengthened administration's relationship with the board.

Critical factors for success included strong board support for the CEO and administration; a willingness to share that trust with the physician panel, realizing that the panel would act in everyone's best interest; the selection of effective cochairs; the physician member commitment; 100 percent transparency; initial "wins"; and the implementation of recommendations. Reid and Allyn conclude, "Your biggest physician critics have the most to gain from this process—engage them and empower physicians to help you navigate medical staff politics" (Allyn, Werft, and Warden 2008).

DEVELOPING THE RIGHT STRATEGIES

The physician strategic plan is based on the organization's strategic priorities, as identified through the integrated strategic financial planning process. Specialty-by-specialty analyses that benefit from physician input provide the sub-plan building blocks for the overall physician strategy. The hospital's strategic planning and financial planning staffs should work together to address the strategic and financial impacts of growth and physician engagement options. The development of a primary care strategy should be a top priority.

Example: Primary Care Network

A hospital is proposing to expand its service area and establish itself as a regional referral center for key programs and services. The hospital is in a strong financial position, capable of funding strategic growth initiatives and investing in additional network/ infrastructure improvements.

Based on a thorough market analysis, the hospital's integrated strategic financial plan identifies the need to deepen and broaden its primary care network to draw patients to the hospital. Core action items selected for developing such a network include the following:

- Develop a hospitalist program to enhance the productivity

and geographic reach of the hospital's PCPs.

- Develop regional referral patterns and relationships.
- Actively add PCPs on an ongoing basis, with a target of 22 physicians during a four- to-five-year period. This strategy would involve bringing new physicians to the area and converting existing physicians who currently refer to other hospitals.

The hospital thoroughly considers likely competitor response to each action item and devises plans to address such responses. Figure 4.2 outlines the hospital's expected capital investment requirements for physician practice support, office space,

Figure 4.2. Financial Requirements and Expected Volume for Primary Care Network

	2007	2008	2009	2010	2011	2012	2013	2014	2015	2016
Physician Additions										
County										
A	2	4	4	–	–	–	–	–	–	–
B	–	4	4	–	–	–	–	–	–	–
C	–	–	2	2	–	–	–	–	–	–
Total	2	8	10	2	–	–	–	–	–	–
Volume										
Inpatient										
Year 1	100	400	500	100	0	0	0	0	0	0
Year 2	0	120	480	600	120	0	0	0	0	0
Year 3 and Ongoing	0	0	120	600	1,200	1,320	1,320	1,320	1,320	1,320
Total	100	520	1,100	1,300	1,320	1,320	1,320	1,320	1,320	1,320
Outpatient	800	4,160	8,800	10,400	10,560	10,560	10,560	10,560	10,560	10,560
Expense ($000s)										
Year 1	$300	$1,240	$1,600	$330	$0	$0	$0	$0	$0	$0
Year 2	0	206	848	1,090	224	0	0	0	0	0
Year 3 and Ongoing	0	0	128	660	1,360	1,540	1,584	1,628	1,672	1,716
Office Space	50	260	540	616	638	660	682	704	726	748
Hospitalist Program	200	400	412	424	437	450	464	478	492	507
Total	$550	$2,106	$3,528	$3,120	$2,659	$2,650	$2,730	$2,810	$2,890	$2,971

Source: Kaufman, Hall & Associates, Inc. Used with permission.

and the hospitalist program. It also includes projections related to the primary care network development. These data are then rolled into the hospital's comprehensive integrated strategic financial plan that outlines all growth initiatives.

Example: A Cardiovascular Center of Excellence

This same hospital targets the development of a highly integrated cardiovascular center of excellence, which is capable of regional draw, as another strategic growth priority. To achieve its goal, the hospital identifies that it will need to accomplish the following:

- Integrate existing stand-alone cardiovascular programs. A paid physician leadership position (medical directorship) at the program level will be created and

internal referral patterns will need to be solidified.

- Extend program reach. This will be accomplished by developing regional referral relationships (referral coaching will be provided), physician outreach, and program-specific marketing initiatives.
- Recruit and ramp up with five additional physicians.
- Establish dedicated inpatient space and resources, including nursing teams, surgical teams, and other resources.
- Reinforce the core program with disease management and wellness promotion.

Figure 4.3 shows the capital investment requirements and volume projections for this strategy. Again, these data are rolled into the hospital's comprehensive integrated strategic financial plan, which identifies

Figure 4.3. Financial Requirements and Expected Volume for Cardiovascular Center of Excellence

	2007	2008	2009	2010	2011	2012	2013	2014	2015	2016
Physician Additions	2	1	1	1	–	–	–	–	–	–
Volume										
Inpatient	150	325	500	650	725	750	750	750	750	750
Outpatient	1,200	2,600	4,000	5,200	5,800	6,000	6,000	6,000	6,000	6,000
Investment Requirement ($000s)	$925	$813	$731	$752	$422	$319	$328	$338	$348	$359

Source: Kaufman, Hall & Associates, Inc. Used with permission.

the financial implications of the total capital investment requirements and volume-based revenue projections.

Figure 4.4 is a consolidated view of the incremental capital required for physician strategy–based growth initiatives. When combined with re-lated revenue projections, the hospital determines whether the projected financial performance supports the proposed capital requirement while maintaining the hospital's liquidity (days cash on hand) and debt capacity targets.

Figure 4.4. Capital Requirements for Growth Initiatives

	2007	2008	2009	2010	2011	2012	2013	2014	2015	2016	Cumulative Total
Investment Requirements ($000s)											
Practice Establishment											
Primary Care	$150	$723	$1,128	$931	$724	$700	$720	$740	$760	$780	$7,356
Cardiac	600	515	424	437	112	0	0	0	0	0	2,088
Orthopedics/Spine	300	412	478	221	174	180	186	192	198	204	2,545
Cancer	0	927	954	545	316	280	288	296	304	312	4,222
General Surgery	0	258	345	355	83	0	0	0	0	0	1,041
Psychology/ Geropsychology	0	103	158	108	112	116	120	124	128	132	1,101
Gastroenterology	250	593	158	0	0	0	0	0	0	0	1,001
Pulmonary	0	258	79	0	0	0	0	0	337	0	674
Subtotal	**$1,300**	**$3,789**	**$3,724**	**$2,597**	**$1,521**	**$1,276**	**$1,314**	**$1,352**	**$1,727**	**$1,428**	**$20,028**
Hospitalist Program	$200	$400	$412	$424	$437	$450	$464	$478	$492	$507	$4,264
Office Space	25	130	243	280	290	300	310	320	330	340	2,568
Leadership Compensation	240	371	382	393	405	417	430	443	456	470	4,007
Outreach	150	309	318	328	337	348	358	369	380	391	3,288
Marketing	155	236	243	251	258	266	274	282	290	299	2,554
Referral Coaching	100	120	60	30	0	0	0	0	0	0	310
Total Incremental Nonfacility Capital	**$2,170**	**$5,355**	**$5,382**	**$4,303**	**$3,248**	**$3,057**	**$3,150**	**$3,244**	**$3,675**	**$3,435**	**$37,019**
Imaging Center	0	0	8,023	0	0	0	0	0	0	0	$8,023
Ambulatory Surgery Center	0	0	0	7,614	0	0	0	0	0	0	7,614
Total Incremental Investment	**$2,170**	**$5,355**	**$13,405**	**$11,917**	**$3,248**	**$3,057**	**$3,150**	**$3,244**	**$3,675**	**$3,435**	**$52,656**

Source: Kaufman, Hall & Associates, Inc. Used with permission.

Example: Ambulatory Surgery Joint Venture

A different hospital that wishes to expand its geographic reach in a selected market targets an ambulatory surgical services center as a strategic growth priority (HFMA 2006). Hospital leaders evaluate a number of options to meet this goal:

- Develop the center or buy a center as a hospital-owned operation.
- Develop the center through a joint venture with physicians.
- Develop the center or buy into a center in partnership with a regional or national ambulatory surgery center operator.
- Develop the center or buy into a center through some combination of the second and third options.

The preliminary planning revolves around a "make versus buy" approach. The organization needs to determine whether new center development is possible given the regulatory environment, space and site considerations, and costs and timing. Data and analyses critical to the decision-making process include market definition, demographic analysis, competitive analysis, physician analysis, service line/specialty analysis, capacity analysis, demand/utilization projections, and financial impact.

An evaluation of the business or financial issues involved in pursuing the ambulatory surgical strategy as a joint venture includes a close look at the cost and benefit of proceeding (or not) with the venture; the investment, ownership, and control provisions; venture structure, financing, and management; and other considerations. The evaluation of these issues must occur within the organization's overall assessment of capital investment opportunities.

A preliminary business assessment of a joint venture provides a sense for whether the venture is going to succeed based on industry, market, financial, and organization-specific factors. Financial analysis at this stage includes return on investment (ROI), net present value, and payback components based on high-level projections.

A thorough review of the costs and benefits of *not* pursuing the joint venture is equally critical. Organizations should carefully quantify the business volume that might be at risk by not entering into a joint venture for an ambulatory surgery center or other venture. Also important is to consider whether there are other physician groups that could be "brought into the hospital's camp" to establish alternative ventures.

The expected ROI of the joint venture should be well defined. This requires realistic projections of utilization/service volumes, development of payment assumptions, and a complete picture of operational, legal, and other costs.

SETTING AND IMPLEMENTING STRATEGIC DIRECTION

Decision making about physician and other organizational strategies occurs within the overall planning process, which takes an integrated look at the "layered effect" of a portfolio of strategies.

For example, Figure 4.5 shows how a hospital considering a new facility and various physician strategies assesses the combined volume impact. The hospital notes that projected volume growth is dependent on both the physician strategy and the new facility.

The hospital takes a close look at the combined incremental cost and volume implications of an aggressive physician strategy, which involves

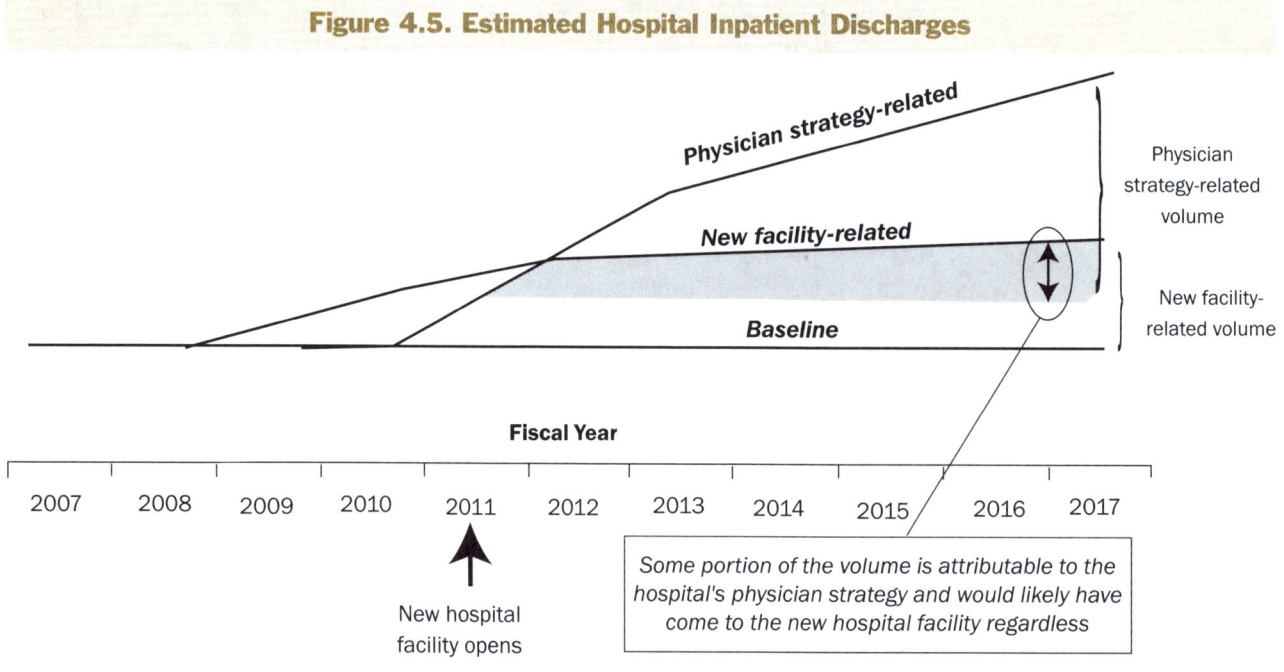

Figure 4.5. Estimated Hospital Inpatient Discharges

Physician strategy-related

New facility-related

Baseline

Physician strategy-related volume

New facility-related volume

Fiscal Year

2007   2008   2009   2010   2011   2012   2013   2014   2015   2016   2017

New hospital facility opens

Some portion of the volume is attributable to the hospital's physician strategy and would likely have come to the new hospital facility regardless

Source: Kaufman, Hall & Associates, Inc. Used with permission.

significant recruitment and employment costs, and the financial impact of financing a replacement facility. The analysis indicates that achieving the physician recruitment plan and length-of-stay targets would be essential. Even with success on the physician front, however, the hospital could not support this magnitude of investment at the level of financial performance expected at its current credit rating.

Hospital leaders return to the "drawing board" to reshape a portfolio of strategies that would ensure both a competitive market position and continued financial success.

Once a potential portfolio is identified, requests for capital related to the portfolio, both as individual initiatives and as a whole, should be evaluated through the organization-wide capital allocation process. This process has specific financial metrics or criteria, as defined by the organization, such as net present value, internal rate of return, payback period, annual return on capital, and annual return on equity. Without such criteria, strategies or initiatives run the risk of being approved on a subjective, political, or first come-first served basis rather than on their ability to meet the organization's strategic and financial objectives.

The portfolio approach to capital investment ensures that investment needs related to physician strategies are balanced with other capital needs. With approval of the selected portfolio of strategies, organizations must commit the capital needed to achieve the plan's success and ensure that the plan is properly implemented and monitored. They also must revisit the plan on a regular (at least annual) basis.

Successful healthcare organizations define indicators of success, measure performance against these indicators, and devise and implement plans to respond to less-than-anticipated performance. Performance indicators for physician strategies and all other strategies, whether focused on financial, quality, market share, satisfaction, or some other metric, must be specific, measurable, attainable, relevant, and time-bound. And they must be used on a regular basis.

Figure 4.6 shows how one health system monitored and measured its success with new strategies in cardiology, spine surgery, and orthopedic surgery.

Accountability is critical. Hospitals should develop a formal process for managing physician engagement initiatives and assign primary

Figure 4.6. Monitoring and Measuring Success of Physician Strategies

	Actual				Projected				Variance			
	Q1	Q2	Q3	Q4	Q1	Q2	Q3	Q4	Q1	Q2	Q3	Q4
Market Share and Utilization												
Service Area Market Share	35.8	36.2	36.3		33	33	33		2.8	3.2	3.3	
Target Cluster 1 Market Share	66.2	66	65.3		65	65	65		1.2	1	0.3	
Target Cluster 2 Market Share	12.3	12.2	11.9		15	15	15		-2.7	-2.8	-3.1	
Visits	12,636	12,551	12,442		12,500	12,500	12,500		136	51	-58	
Surgeries	2,589	2,421	2,211		2,500	2,500	2,500		89	-79	-289	
Program/Service Development												
Cardiology Procedures	643	660	684		575	575	575		68	85	109	
Catheterization Laboratory Procedures	881	911	988		850	850	850		31	61	138	
Spine Surgeries	88	90	75		125	125	125		-37	-35	-50	
Orthopedic Surgeries	390	420	360		400	400	400		-10	20	-40	
Operations												
Expense per Adjusted Day	804	866	893		775	775	775		29	91	118	
Compensation Ratio	52.1	54	55		50	50	50		2.1	4	5	
Average Length of Stay	5.3	5.6	5.6		5.9	5.9	5.9		-0.6	-0.3	-0.3	
Finance												
Days Cash on Hand	144	140	135		150	150	150		-6	-10	-15	
Operating Margin	2.2	2	1.6		2.5	2.5	2.5		-0.3	-0.5	-0.9	
Earnings Before Interest, Depreciation, and Amortization Margin	9.5	9.3	9		10	10	10		-0.5	-0.7	-1	
Debt Service Coverage	2.8	2.7	2.6		3	3	3		-0.2	-0.3	-0.4	

Source: Kaufman, Hall & Associates, Inc. Used with permission.

and supporting accountabilities to leadership—starting with the CEO—and staff.

CONCLUDING COMMENTS

Executives of successful organizations take a proactive approach to engaging physicians, recognizing that strong hospital-physician relations are critical to the sustainable growth required for ongoing competitive performance. The strength of relationships with physicians influences the hospital's ability to recruit top physicians and staff, achieve quality initiatives, and meet patient needs in both inpatient and outpatient arenas.

Current Realities Related to Physician Strategies

1. The age dichotomy is real:
   - Experienced physicians are focused on preserving historical income levels that are under pressure.
   - Younger physicians are focused on managing risk and maintaining lifestyle.
   - Hospitals must find strategies to appeal to both.
2. Opportunities for collaboration vary by clinical specialty:
   - There is no one-size-fits-all answer.
   - Legal/financial alternatives to align with PCPs are limited.
3. There truly is strength in numbers:
   - Where physicians have organized, they are more powerful.
   - Where larger groups of physicians are teamed with hospitals, both are stronger.
4. Geography matters:
   - Payer mix and patient mix, which vary by geographic location, affect organizational and physician practice profitability.
   - Whether a hospital exists in a competitive market or is a sole provider has significant impact on the development and success of physician-hospital engagement strategies.
   - Attractiveness of the hospital's geographic location to new physicians enhances recruitment initiatives.
5. Creating the best "workshop" is still critical for differentiation:
   - Hospitals must ensure the quality of affiliated specialists.
   - Advanced IT, including EHR/EMR, is required for the hospital of the future.
   - Well-trained, easy-to-work-with support staff will enhance physician satisfaction and retention.
   - Efficient operating rooms increase physician and staff productivity and satisfaction and hospital throughput.
   - Hospital-based physicians, including hospitalists, intensivists, radiologists, anesthesiologists, emergency physicians, and pathologists, enhance care quality and efficiency.
   - Administrators who communicate effectively and follow through on promises are key to physician satisfaction.
6. Capital still rules:
   - The have and have-not hospitals will deploy different strategies.
   - The haves will win in competitive markets because they can invest more and sustain bigger losses if necessary.

Source: Kaufman, Hall & Associates, Inc. Used with permission.

Ultimately, hospitals and physicians share the six goals for healthcare articulated by the Institute of Medicine, namely healthcare that is safe, effective, timely, equitable, efficient, and patient-centered (IOM 2001). How to get there represents the challenge. There is no tried and true physician engagement plan that works for all organizations or all physicians. Rather, hospital leaders must work closely with physicians to develop organization-specific, service line-specific, and market-specific plans; test and refine these plans during implementation; and revise the plans through the years to reflect current realities. At press time, six realities warrant mention (Sidebar 4.2), but stay tuned—others will develop. So read the literature; and, most of all, keep talking with physicians.

Bibliography

Allyn, T. R., R. Werft, and J. C. Warden. 2008. "Medical Advisory Panels: A Model for Collaboration." Presented at the Physician Strategies Summit, Los Angeles, March 3.

Allyn, T. R. 2008. Personal communication, Aug. 26, 2008.

American College of Healthcare Executives (ACHE). 2008. "Top Issues Confronting Hospitals: 2007." *Healthcare Executive*, March/April: 84–85.

American College of Physicians. 2006. "Internal Medicine Residency Match Results and Survey of Residents' Future Career Plans Underscores Need for Comprehensive Reform." Press release, March 16.

American Medical Association. 2007. *Physician Characteristics and Distribution in the U.S.* Chicago: American Medical Association.

Andrews, B. W. 2007. "The Carilion Clinic: Transforming a Health System to Meet the Quality Mandate." Presentation at the Fourth Annual Conference on Physician Agreements and Ventures, Chicago, Nov.

Association of American Medical Colleges. 2006. *AAMC Statement on the Physician Workforce*, June. [Online information; retrieved 8/08.] www.aamc.org/workforce/workforceposition.pdf.

———. 2007a. "Medical Student Education: Cost, Debt, and Resident Stipend Facts." [Online information; retrieved 5/08.] www.aamc.org/programs/first/debtfactcard.pdf.

———. 2007b. *Recent Studies and Reports on Physician Shortages in the U.S.* Washington, DC: Center for Workforce Studies. [Online report; retrieved 3/08.] www.aamc.org/workforce/recent-workforcestudies2007.pdf.

———. 2008. *Addressing Healthcare Workforce Issues for the Future.* Testimony presented before the Committee on Health, Education, Labor, and Pensions of the U.S. Senate by Edward Salsberg, MPA, director of AAMC's Center for Workforce Studies, Feb. 12. [Online information; retrieved 8/08.] www.aamc.org/advocacy/library/workforce/testimony/2008/021208.pdf.

Bader, B. S., E. A. Kazemek, P. R. Knecht, and R. W. Witalis. 2008. "Physicians on the Board: Conflict over Conflicts." *BoardRoom Press*, Feb.

Berenson, R. A., P. B. Ginsburg, and J. H. May. 2006. "Hospital-Physician Relations: Cooperation, Competition, or Separation?" *Health Affairs*, Web Exclusive, Dec. 5. [Online information; retrieved 7/08.] http://content.healthaffairs.org/cgi/content/abstract/hlthaff.26.1.w31.

Blaszyk, M. D., and J. Hill-Mischell. 2007. *Joint Ventures: From Policy to Post-Execution Monitoring*. Skokie, IL: Kaufman, Hall & Associates, Inc.

Blesch, G. "Not So Taxing After All." *Modern Healthcare*, Oct. 29.

Brierton, J. 2004. "Medical Malpractice Captive Insurance Company." Office of Legislative Research Report. [Online report; retrieved 3/08.] www.cga.ct.gov/2004/rpt/2004-R-0408.htm.

Centers for Medicare & Medicaid Services. 2007. "CMS Revises Payment Structure for Ambulatory Surgical Centers and Proposes Policy and Payment Changes for Hospital Outpatient." Press Release dated July 16, 2007. [Online information; retrieved 8/22/08.] www.cms.hhs.gov.

Cohen, R. L. undated. *Physician-Hospital Joint Venture and Affiliation Models*. Omaha, NE: Kutak Rock.

Cohn, K. H. 2005. *Better Communication for Better Care: Mastering Physician-Administrator Collaboration*. Chicago: Health Administration Press.

———. 2006. *Collaborate for Success! Breakthrough Strategies for Engaging Physicians*. Chicago: Health Administration Press.

Cohn, K. H., T. R. Allyn, and R. A. Reid. 2006. "Structured Dialogue Between Physicians and Administrators Yields Positive Results." *Physician Executive* 32 (4): 22–25.

Cortese, D., and R. Smoldt. 2006. "Taking Steps Toward Integration." *Health Affairs*, web exclusive, Dec. 5. [Online article; retrieved 7/08.] http://content.healthaffairs.org/cgi/content/abstract/hlthaff.26.1.w68.

Council on Physician and Nurse Supply. 2007. *2007 National Physician and Nurse Supply Survey*. Philadelphia, PA: Council on Physician and Nurse Supply.

Davis, J. M. 2007. "The MOB Outbreak." *CIRE Magazine*, March–April.

Fitch Ratings. 2006. *Quality and Patient Safety Spending in the Not-for-Profit Hospital Sector*. Special Report. New York: Fitch Ratings.

———. 2007. *Understanding Hospital-Physician Alignment*. Special Report. New York: Fitch Ratings.

Goldsmith, J. 2006. "Hospitals and Physicians: Not A Pretty Picture." *Health Affairs,* web exclusive, Dec. 5. [Online article; retrieved 7/08.] http://content.healthaffairs.org/cgi/content/abstract/hlthaff.26.1.w72.

Goldstein, L. 2007. "Rating Agency Insights: Hospital-Physician Integration." *Kaufman Hall Report*, Spring.

The Governance Institute. 2007a. *Boards × 4. Governance Structures and Practices: The 2007 Biennial Survey of Hospitals and Healthcare Systems.* San Diego, CA: The Governance Institute.

———. 2007b. *Emerging Models for Physician-Hospital Alignment.* CEO Roundtable. San Diego, CA: The Governance Institute.

Grossman, J. M., T. S. Bodenheimer, and K. McKenzie. 2006. "Hospital-Physician Portals: The Role of Competition in Driving Clinical Data Exchange." *Health Affairs* 25 (6): 1629–1635.

Grube, M. E. 2007. "Growing the Top Line: 5 Strategies to Expand Your Business." *hfm*, May.

Grube, M. E., R. S. Gish, and S. N. Tkach. 2008. "Achieving Scale: Strategies for Sustained Competitive Performance." *hfm*, May.

Healthcare Financial Management Association (HFMA). 2005. *Strategies for Effective Capital Structure Management.* Financing the Future II Series. Westchester, IL: HFMA.

———. 2006. *Joint Ventures with Physicians and Other Partners.* Financing the Future II Series. Westchester, IL: HFMA.

Inglehart, J. K. 2008. "Grassroots Activism and the Pursuit of an Expanded Physician Supply." *New England Journal of Medicine* 358 (16): 1741–1748.

Institute of Medicine (IOM). 2001. *Crossing the Quality Chasm: A New Health System for the 21st Century.* Washington, DC: National Academies Press.

Johnson, B., and D. Walker Keegan. 2006. *Physician Compensation Plans: State-of-the-Art Strategies.* Englewood, CO: Medical Group Management Association.

Kaufman, K. 2006. *Best Practice Financial Management: Six Key Concepts for Healthcare Leaders,* 3rd ed. Chicago: Health Administration Press.

Kilo, C. M., and M. Leavitt. 2005. *Medical Practice Transformation with Information Technology.* Chicago: Healthcare Information Management and Systems Society.

Lindenauer, P. K., M. B. Rothberg, P. S. Pekow, C. Kenwood, E. M. Benjamin, and A. D. Auerbach. 2007. "Outcomes of Care by Hospitalists, General Internists, and Family Physicians." *New England Journal of Medicine* 357 (25): 2589–2600.

McGowan, R. A., and A. S. MacNulty. 2005. "Strategies for Strengthening Physician-Hospital Alignment: A National Study." Noblis (formerly Mitretek Systems, Inc.). Chicago: Society for Healthcare Strategy and Market Development.

Medical Group Management Association (MGMA). 2007. *Cost Survey: 2007 Report Based on 2006 Data.* Englewood, CO: MGMA.

———. 2007. *Management Compensation Survey: 2007 Report Based on 2006 Data.* Englewood, CO: MGMA.

———. 2007. *Physician Compensation and Production Survey: 2007 Report Based on 2006 Data.* Englewood, CO: MGMA.

Medicare Payment Advisory Commission. 2008. *A Data Book: Healthcare Spending and the Medicare Program.* Washington, DC: Medicare Payment Advisory Commission.

Mello, M. M. 2006. *Understanding Medical Malpractice Insurance: A Primer.* Princeton, NJ: The Robert Wood Johnson Foundation.

Merritt Hawkins & Associates. 2007. "2007 Physician Inpatient/Outpatient Revenue Survey." [Online information; retrieved 3/08.] http://www.merritthawkins.com/pdf/2007_Physician_Inpatient_Outpatient_Revenue_Survey.pdf.

Moody's Investors Service. 2007. *Designing the Healthcare Delivery System of the Future.* Special Comment. New York: Moody's Investors Service.

Orlikoff, J. E., and M. K. Totten. 2005. "Physicians in Governance: The Board's New Challenge." *Trustee,* July/Aug.

Patel, A. D., A.M. Khorover, and J.J. Pizzo. 2007. *Hospital-Physician Strategic Ventures.* San Diego, CA: The Governance Institute.

Pham, H. H., and P. B. Ginsburg. 2007. "Unhealthy Trends: The Future of Physician Services." *Health Affairs* 26 (6): 1586–1598.

Rosenfield, R. 2005. As cited in HFMA. *Financing the Future II.* 2005. *Strategies for Effective Capital Structure Management.* Westchester, IL: Healthcare Financial Management Association.

St. Luke's Health Initiatives and Arizona Hospital and Healthcare Association. 2005. *Arizona Health Futures: Can This Marriage Be Saved? Physician-Hospital Relationships.* Phoenix, AZ: St. Luke's Health Initiatives.

Standard & Poor's. 2007. *Evolving Physician Relations Continue to Affect U.S. Not-for-Profit Health Care Credit.* New York: Standard & Poor's.

Starfield, B., and G. E. Fryer, Jr. 2007. "The Primary Care Physician Workforce: Ethical and Policy Implications." *Annals of Family Medicine* 5 (6): 486–491.

Sussman, J. H. 2007. *The Healthcare Executive's Guide to Allocating Capital.* Chicago: Health Administration Press.

Tu, H. T., and P. B. Ginsburg. 2006. *Losing Ground: Physician Income, 1995–2003.* Tracking Report 15. Washington, DC: Center for Studying Health System Change.

Tu, H. T., and A. S. O'Malley. 2007. *Exodus of Male Physicians from Primary Care Drives Shift to Specialty Practice.* Tracking Report 17. Washington, DC: Center for Studying Health System Change.

Wachter, R. M. 2004. "Physician–Hospital Alignment: The Elusive Ingredient." The Commonwealth Fund, July. [Online commentary; retrieved 7/08.] http://www.commonwealthfund.org/publications/publications_show.htm?doc_id = 235208.

Warden, J. C., and K. Woodward. 2008. "Creating a Sustainable Physician Strategy." *hfm,* Jan.

York, R., and J. Benjamin. 2008. "Are Your Demand Projections Grounded in Market Realities?" *Strategic Financial Planning Newsletter,* Winter.

U. S. Department of Health and Human Services. 2006. *Physician Supply and Demand: Projections to 2020.* Washington, DC: Health Resources and Services Administration.

About the Author

Jay C. Warden, senior vice president of Kaufman, Hall & Associates, Inc., has more than 20 years of healthcare management experience. He has held senior leadership positions in hospitals and health systems, medical groups, physician management organizations, consulting firms, and software companies.

As a member of Kaufman Hall's strategy practice, Mr. Warden assists hospitals and health systems with integrated strategic and financial planning, strategic market assessments, and business development/market growth strategies. He also leads Kaufman Hall's medical staff planning and physician strategy practice.

Prior to joining Kaufman Hall, Mr. Warden was president of Sg2 Consulting, where he led the firm's strategy consulting practice. His previous experience includes strategy consulting experience at Tiber Group (now Navigant) and system and hospital leadership roles with a large hospital/health system.

Mr. Warden received his bachelor's degree from Dartmouth College and his master's degrees in business administration and health services administration from the University of Michigan.

Acknowledgments

Special thanks for making this book possible are due to many people. First, thank you to the executives of client healthcare organizations, whose ideas and practical applications of high-quality physician strategies have greatly enriched this book. Second, many colleagues at Kaufman, Hall & Associates have greatly contributed to this book. Partners Kenneth Kaufman, Mark E. Grube, and Jason H. Sussman deserve special mention for their work through the decades in combining strategy and finance for organizational direction-setting. This approach, described in the context of physician strategy direction-setting in this book, has helped hundreds of hospitals and health systems achieve sustainable competitive performance. Thanks also to Nancy G. Haiman, publisher of Kaufman Hall's Learning Division, for her skill and oversight as editor of this book. Last, and certainly not least, many thanks to my family for their love and support through, and in spite of, my many professional activities that have spilled into family time. Everything I do, whether at work or at home, would be impossible without them.